The Sciences of Animal Welfare

The Universities Federation for Animal Welfare

UFAW, founded 1926, is an internationally recognized, independent, scientific and educational animal welfare charity concerned with promoting high standards of welfare for farm, companion, laboratory and captive wild animals, and for those animals with which we interact in the wild. It works to improve animals' lives by:

- Promoting and supporting developments in the science and technology that underpin advances in animal welfare;

- Promoting education in animal care and welfare;

- Providing information, organising meetings, and publishing books, videos, articles, technical reports and the journal *Animal Welfare*;

- Providing expert advice to government departments and other bodies and helping to draft and amend laws and guidelines;

- Enlisting the energies of animal keepers, scientists, veterinarians, lawyers and others who care about animals.

"Improvements in the care of animals are not now likely to come of their own accord, merely by wishing them: there must be research ... and it is in sponsoring research of this kind, and making its results widely known, that UFAW performs one of its most valuable services."

Sir Peter Medawar CBE FRS, 8th May 1957
Nobel Laureate (1960), Chairman of the UFAW Scientific Advisory Committee (1951–1962)

UFAW relies on the generosity of the public through legacies and donations to carry out its work improving the welfare of animal now and in the future. For further information about UFAW and how you can help promote and support its work, please contact us at the address below.

Universities Federation for Animal Welfare
The Old School, Brewhouse Hill, Wheathampstead, Herts AL4 8AN, UK
Tel: 01582 831818 Fax: 01582 831414 Website: www.ufaw.org.uk
Email: ufaw@ufaw.org.uk

The Sciences of Animal Welfare

David J. Mellor
Professor of Animal Welfare Science,
Professor of Applied Physiology and Bioethics,
Co-Director, Animal Welfare Science and
Bioethics Centre,
Massey University, Palmerston North, New Zealand

Emily Patterson-Kane
Animal Welfare Scientist,
American Veterinary Medical Association,
Schaumburg, IL, USA

Kevin J. Stafford
Professor of Veterinary Ethology,
Co-Director, Animal Welfare Science and
Bioethics Centre,
Massey University, Palmerston North, New Zealand

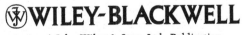

WILEY-BLACKWELL

A John Wiley & Sons, Ltd., Publication

This edition first published 2009
© 2009 by UFAW

Series editors
James K. Kirkwood and Robert C. Hubrecht
Wiley-Blackwell is an imprint of John Wiley & Sons, formed by the merger of Wiley's global
Scientific, Technical and Medical business with Blackwell Publishing.

Editorial offices
9600 Garsington Road, Oxford, OX4 2DQ, United Kingdom
2121 State Avenue, Ames, Iowa 50014-8300, USA

For details of our global editorial offices, for customer services and for information about
how to apply for permission to reuse the copyright material in this book please see our website
at www.wiley.com/wiley-blackwell.

Library of Congress Cataloging-in-Publication Data
Mellor, David J.
    The sciences of animal welfare / David J. Mellor, Emily Patterson-Kane, Kevin J. Stafford.
        p. ; cm. -- (UFAW animal welfare series)
    Includes bibliographical references and index.
    ISBN 978-1-4051-3495-8 (pbk. : alk. paper) 1. Animal welfare. 2. Veterinary medicine. 3.
Agriculture. I. Patterson-Kane, Emily. II. Stafford, Kevin J. III. Universities Federation for Animal
Welfare. IV. Title. V. Series: UFAW animal welfare series.
    [DNLM: 1. Animal Welfare. 2. Animal Use Alternatives--methods. 3. Behavior, Animal. 4. Pain--
veterinary. 5. Veterinary Medicine--methods. HV 4708 M527s 2009]

HV4708.M45 2009

636.08'32--dc22

                                                        2009016432

A catalogue record for this book is available from the British Library.

Set in 10/12.5 pt Sabon by Newgen Imaging Systems Pvt. Ltd, Chennai, India

1 2009

Contents

Foreword

From the Universities Federation for Animal Welfare's (UFAW's) very first meeting in 1926 at Birkbeck College in London, the organisation's aim has been to harness the power of science for the benefit of animals' welfare. This was expressed in the rather indigestible original wording of one of its two objectives, which is: 'To encourage and promote, through the process of education, good management and husbandry practices whereby the needs of animals are properly understood and met, and, in advancement thereof, to contribute to the store of scientific knowledge by funding and engaging in animal welfare research and by publishing the results thereof.'

As David Mellor, Emily Patterson Kane and Kevin Stafford make clear in this wide-ranging, fascinating and thought-provoking book, there are many scientific challenges to be addressed in tackling the multitude of pressing animal welfare problems of which we are aware and in attaining a proper understanding of animals' needs and how these can be met. Although much has been learned already in some fields, for a good, shared, science-based understanding of the needs of all the species we keep, or with which we interact, there is still a long way to go. As the book neatly outlines, attitudes to animals vary greatly among cultures and between individuals, and have changed with time. Inventing and designing practical scientific approaches to assess the importance to animals of various aspects (present or absent) of their environments often requires great ingenuity. Sharp and open minds are needed and, as the authors also intimate, drawing clear conclusions from the findings can sometimes be much less straightforward than was foreseen. However, despite the difficulties of the terrain, the book provides many instructive examples of how scientific approaches have been able to inform policy decisions regarding aspects of the handling, keeping and humane killing of animals.

I am most grateful to the authors for this excellent contribution to the UFAW/ Wiley-Blackwell Animal Welfare Series.

James K. Kirkwood
May 2009

Preface

It is only since the early to mid-1990s that animal welfare science has emerged as a recognized discipline with dedicated degree courses, textbooks, journals, research departments and specialists. Much of the present content of animal welfare science therefore rests on foundations laid over many previous decades by behavioural, nutritional, livestock, physiological, veterinary and other animal-based sciences. Initial application of established methodologies led to substantial advances in understanding relevant to animal welfare, although at that time the ideas were only beginning to be framed in those terms. These advances in their turn gave impetus to innovative methodological developments and further improvements in knowledge within the animal welfare science arena itself, thereby enhancing the credibility of its claim to be a discipline in its own right.

It is understandable that with the emergence of a new discipline its adherents would wish to enhance its standing by encouraging publication of research findings and scholarly comment in newly formed or relevant existing journals. Animal welfare scientists are no exception. Publishing in journals such as *Animal Welfare*, first issued by the Universities Federation for Animal Welfare in 1992, and in the behavioural, laboratory animal and veterinary sciences literature, enables research and other articles on welfare-related topics to be located easily, which is an advantage. But this can also restrict the scope of reading on the subject, and that would be a disadvantage if it precluded an outward-looking perspective and familiarity with orientations and publications from other disciplines. Thus, although animal welfare science is now an established discipline, its future vitality will depend on continuing external contibutions from its progenitor disciplines and from others. Accordingly, we, the authors, advocate a multi-disciplinary approach. A key theme of this book, therefore, is that by operating widely within diverse disciplines, and perhaps more importantly, at the margins between disciplines, fresh insights can be obtained which will enliven thinking and improve animal welfare; hence the title of our book with its focus on the *sciences* of animal welfare, not the *science* of animal welfare. We have provided several examples of the benefits of this open thinking.

The many decades of research and scholarship in the disciplines that underpin much of the present content of animal welfare science also provided it with a history of substantial successes, as well as some problems. In current advocacy for animals, it often appears that the successes are ignored or conveniently forgotten, and the problems highlighted. Some animal advocates appear reluctant to give credit to scientists and others for their good intentions and for making improvements in animal welfare, because to do so may appear to undermine the strength of the advocates' assertions that animal welfare in general, or in regard to a particular problem, is currently deplorable and requires urgent attention. Alternatively, given that numerous major advances in knowledge were made decades ago and solved or substantially alleviated the problems to which they were applied, there may simply be no current memory or direct experience of what was then commonplace and what, if found today, would indeed be strongly deplored. Another theme of this book, therefore, is to acknowledge our debt to past successes in animal-based science disciplines, successes that markedly improved animal welfare long before the notion of animal welfare entered common parlance. In doing so, however, we have not sought to play down other problems which then appeared unexpectedly.

It is a truism that people are limited in understanding by their own experience and expectations. This applies equally to everyday life as it does to the present evaluation of animals through the vehicle of animal-based sciences. Thus, for example, if prevailing thinking has it that animals lack feelings and the capacity to suffer at all or in particular respects, or if their cognitive or sensory capabilities are considered to be inferior to or no better than those of people, then the data generated will usually be interpreted in those terms. This has always been the case and would be a recipe for stagnation if no other factors came into play. However, movement in thinking does occur when new information challenges current paradigms sufficiently for them to be modified or discarded, although this rarely occurs without resistance from the creators of, or the strong adherents to, the challenged paradigm. Accordingly, another theme of this book is that there is value in questioning the often-unexamined fundamental assumptions that each person makes about animals and their functional capabilities. The purpose of this is to allow the animals to reveal themselves as they truly are, rather than have them understood only through a straightjacket of limiting presuppositions. We provide examples to show how the resulting refreshed thinking will help to refocus attention on a fundamental feature of what animal welfare represents, namely the animal's own experience of its internal state and of the impact of its environment.

Three of us authored this book. Our experience, although different, is complementary. We see the wider coverage this allowed as positive. We all fully support the content and orientation of the book, which we scoped together and reviewed regularly while writing it. Each of us took responsibility for preparing the first draft of particular chapters, passing them to the others for comment, and one of us (DJM) took the role of coordinating co-author for all chapters. Although all chapters therefore contain contributions from the three of us, the reader will become aware that three distinct voices have remained. This too we see as positive in both providing variety for the reader and in highlighting the writing style of the co-author who prepared the first draft of each chapter.

The book is divided into five sections. The *Introduction* contains one chapter in which we set the scene by outlining our views on a range of issues that are relevant to animal welfare. The section entitled *Paths from the Past* provides historical perspectives. Its three chapters deal in turn with the major improvements made to animal welfare by agricultural sciences, veterinary science and genetics. It acknowledges that some developments also had negative consequences for animals. The two chapters in *Assessment of Animal Welfare* consider grading animal welfare compromise, ways of mitigating suffering, and the strengths and weaknesses of standardized behavioural testing of animals. In the three chapters in the section on *Human Inputs and Animal Welfare,* we consider positive and negative features of human–animal interactions and environmental enrichment, and impacts of societal contexts on animal welfare thinking. The final section, *Thinking Outside the Box*, contains two chapters. In the first, which deals with various aspects of sleep in animals, we show that fresh insights can arise by wide consultation of the scientific literature well beyond that commonly reviewed by animal welfare scientists. In the second chapter, and the last in the book, we very briefly draw attention to the non-science, wider context of animal welfare science. Our purpose is to highlight, in general terms, the diverse interests within society that influence attitudes towards animals and reciprocal opportunities for animal welfare scientists to influence those attitudes. In addition, we note the importance of recognizing that thinking from outside animal welfare science and the related sciences also affects attitudes towards, and the implementation of, practical, regulatory and advisory measures to deal with animal welfare problems.

Throughout we have endeavoured to inform, challenge, refresh and excite the reader. We hope that at the end of each chapter the reader will say 'Well, I didn't know that!,' or 'I had never thought of it that way!,' or 'That's interesting!,' or indeed 'I don't agree with that!' We have used section headings to divide each chapter, but instead of using conventional subheadings we have stated key concepts which we then discuss. This was done to help the reader focus on the issues being explored. To assist the reader further, each chapter begins with a list of the key concepts discussed within each section. This enables the reader to have some foreknowledge of the path the ideas will follow in each chapter before beginning the journey.

We have enjoyed writing this book, and we hope you will enjoy reading it.

David J. Mellor
Emily Patterson-Kane
Kevin J. Stafford
January 2009

Acknowledgements

While writing this book we have each drawn widely on our own life experience, deriving confidence from both its personal and professional dimensions. On the personal side we recognize and gladly acknowledge the unfailing support and encouragement of our families, freely given over many years, and in particular we want to mention Lynda and Thomas Mellor, Jacky Patterson-Kane and Yvonne Stafford.

On the professional paths we each travelled prior to conceiving this book many people influenced us and thereby broadened the experience we collectively drew upon while formulating the ideas we have now presented here. There are far too many to name, but we recognize a huge debt and warmly thank them all. They include academic and professional mentors, science leaders, close work colleagues and friends, collaborating scientists, members of the medical and veterinary professions, postgraduate and undergraduate students, philosophers, ethicists, government regulators, farmers and other animal-based industry personnel, animal welfare advocates and lawyers, animal rights activists, members of other non-governmental organizations, lay people who own and care about animals, and numerous others.

The book itself was further enhanced by direct input from others. We wish to specifically thank Michael Appleby, John Barnett, David Bayvel, Hugh Blair, Michelle Cooke, Mark Fisher, Neville Gregory, Corrin Hulls, Craig Johnson, Roger Lentle, Dave West and Peter Wilson for most helpful discussion and other inputs. In addition, we appreciate the helpful editorial comments on the submitted manuscript provided by Robert Hubrecht and James Kirkwood of UFAW.

We thank the following people in New Zealand for making available their photographs for inclusion in the book: Tamara Diesch, Stokes Valley; Mark Fisher, Kotare Bioethics, Hastings; Mark Oliver, Liggins Institute, University of Auckland; and Dave West, Lois Wilkinson and Andrew Worth, Massey University, Palmerston North. Finally, we thank MAF New Zealand for financially supporting the material completion of the book.

Part 1

Introduction

Focus of Animal Welfare

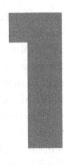

This book is about the way different scientific disciplines contribute to our understanding and management of animal welfare. At the outset we note that particular scientific ideas, once they have been rigorously and systematically formulated and objectively and critically reviewed, do not remain fixed. Rather, they develop continuously as related scientific perspectives and knowledge evolve. Thus, few scientific conclusions remain unaltered for long. In time most are refined, changed markedly or replaced. Moreover, conflicting interpretations of scientific data may arise as particular areas are explored in greater depth or in different ways, so that there may be two or more scientific explanations of a particular phenomenon. Accordingly, there is often no single, immutable interpretation at a scientific-functional level by which issues may be resolved, and judgements need to be based on the weight of scientific evidence for or against particular propositions. Yet the creative tension between alternative explanations of particular phenomena motivates further research and thinking and contributes to the continuing development of the discipline.

These general dynamics apply just as much to animal welfare science as to all other scientific disciplines. Elements of this are illustrated in the following chapters. We will show that various disciplines have contributed to improving animal welfare in the past, and that reference to insights from other disciplines may now redirect thinking about animal welfare in ways that will provide new perspectives on its assessment and management in the future. As a starting point for this some key concepts are outlined briefly to focus thinking in preparation for the chapters that follow.

1.1 Animal Welfare is a Driver for Ethical Behaviour Towards Animals

After many years of reflection, contemporary societies generally hold the view that it is acceptable to use animals for human purposes provided that such use is humane and justified (Banner *et al.*, 1995). It is also recognized that animals can suffer and that it matters to them how they are treated. In using animals for our purposes we exercise varying degrees of control over the quality and duration of their lives. That control gives us the *opportunity* to manage them humanely. Moreover, using them for our own purposes, not theirs, *requires* us to do so. Accordingly, we have an ethical 'duty of care' towards the animals in our control and this translates into a practical obligation to keep their welfare at acceptable levels. To do this we need an understanding of what animal welfare is.

1.2 There is no Single Unified Definition of Animal Welfare

To date, no single unified definition of animal welfare has emerged. This is partly because, at any one time, scientists, scholars and other contributors have emphasized different facets of animal functionality and animal–human or animal–environmental interactions. It is also partly because changes over time in our understanding of the ways animals may experience their functional status or their participation in interactions with people and the environment have drawn attention to limitations in extant definitions. Moreover, when assessing the welfare status of animals in practical contexts different emphasis has been placed on different facets of current definitions (Nordenfelt, 2006). At present, three general orientations can be recognized; they focus largely on biological function, affective state and natural state (Fraser, 2003).

The *biological function* view holds that, in general, welfare is good when the animals are healthy, growing and reproducing well, and, for farm animals in particular, when good meat, milk, egg and fibre productivity of individuals is broadly aligned with good health and reproductive performance (e.g. Barnett and Hemsworth, 2003). The *affective state* orientation emphasizes the potential for animals to suffer or have positive experiences (e.g. Duncan, 1996; Dawkins, 1998). Thus, good welfare is said to be present when an animal adapts without suffering and/or with positive emotional experiences (feelings) during its interactions with other animals, people and the environment. Finally, according to the *natural state* view, an animal's welfare may be compromised in proportion to how far the conditions in which it is kept deviate from the original wild state of the species and, in particular, by the extent to which the animal is or is not able to express most of its natural behaviours (e.g. Rollin, 1992; Alroe *et al.*, 2001).

The outcomes of judgements made about the acceptability or otherwise of the ways we manage animals are likely to differ depending on which of these three orientations is emphasized (Fraser, 2003). They will also depend on how an animal's welfare status may be assessed (Nordenfelt, 2006), for instance in terms of how well it copes with the environment (Broom, 1996), its fitness in terms of survival and reproductive success (Barnard and Hurst, 1996), or whether its needs are being met (Dawkins, 1983). With a needs focus, for instance, understanding animal welfare will depend critically on what an animal's needs are considered to be, and in what ways and to what extent the non-satisfaction of those needs affects the animal adversely (Mellor and Reid, 1994).

1.3 Animal Welfare is a State in an Animal and Requires both Consciousness and Sentience

The welfare status of an animal, whether good, neutral or bad, represents the integrated outcome of all sensory and other neural inputs from within its body and from the environment, inputs which are processed and interpreted by the animal's brain according to its species-specific and individual nature and experience, and then perceived consciously. Accordingly, for an animal to perceive states which we consider reflect its welfare it must be both alive and conscious, and it must also be sentient; that is, it must have a brain of sufficient functional sophistication to transduce sensory inputs into cognitive or emotional experiences it can interpret as good, neutral or bad (Mellor and Reid, 1994; Mellor and Diesch, 2006). This implies that consideration of welfare is limited to higher animals, but it is not clear whether only (or all) vertebrates should be included, and if not, where the line of exclusion should be drawn among the invertebrates (Davie and Kopf, 2006; Kirkwood, 2006; Kendrick, 2007). Within sentient animals, there is also the question of when, during their development from immature to more mature stages, fetal and newborn animals, marsupial pouch young and pre-hatched young of avian and other species become conscious (Mellor and Diesch, 2006, 2007; see also Chapter 10 in this volume).

1.4 Animal Welfare may be Characterized in Terms of Five Domains

Notwithstanding the various definitions of animal welfare and approaches to welfare assessment (see Nordenfelt, 2006), we have found it useful to focus on animals' needs in five domains of potential welfare compromise, and the degree to which those needs are or are not met (Mellor and Reid, 1994; Mellor and Stafford, 2001; Chapter 5). Thus, we recognize nutritional, environmental, health, behavioural and mental domains of welfare, and describe good welfare as existing when an animal's needs in these interacting domains are largely being met (Figure 1.1). We also note that an animal's status can vary on a continuum between high welfare and its opposite of extreme suffering. Accordingly, it is proposed that sensory and other neural inputs associated with the nutritional, environmental, health and behavioural domains (considered to be largely physical or functional), together with additional cognitive inputs, are processed and then express themselves (within the mental domain) in terms of the animal's conscious subjective experience. It is the character of this conscious experience and its associated position on the welfare-suffering continuum which determine the animal's overall welfare status (Mellor and Reid, 1994; Mellor and Stafford, 2001).

PHYSICAL COMPONENTS

Domain 1	Domain 2	Domain 3	Domain 4
Water deprivation, food deprivation, malnutrition	Environmental challenge	Disease, injury functional impairment	Behavioural or interactive restriction

MENTAL COMPONENTS

Domain 5		
Thirst	Debility	Loneliness
Hunger	Weakness	Helplessness
Nausea	Sickness	Boredom
Pain (short-lived)	Pain (moderate)	Pain (persistent, untreatable)
Fear	Breathlessness	Breathlessness (incurable)
Anxiety (transient)	(transient, curable)	Anxiety (persistent)
Frustration (transient)	Dizziness	Frustration (persistent)
		Distress

Animal Welfare Status

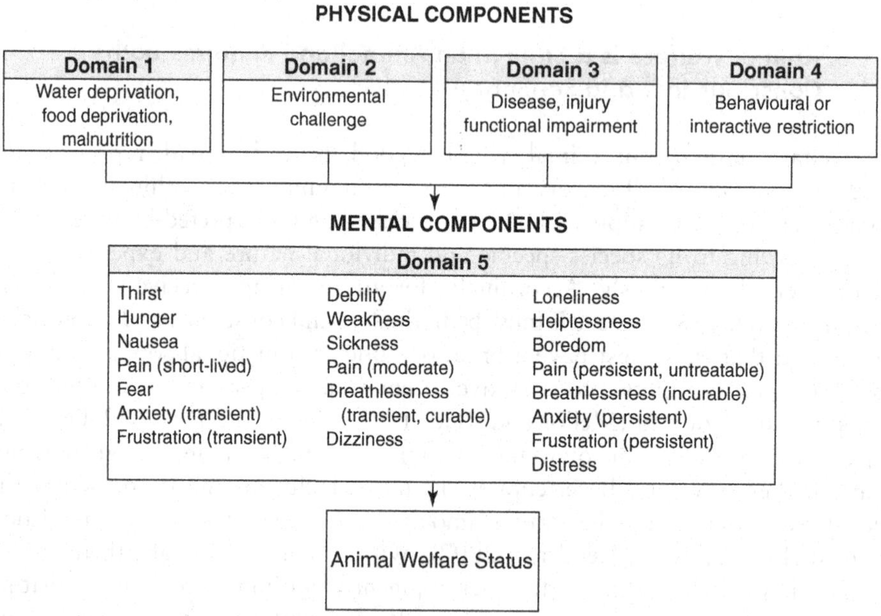

Figure 1.1 The five domains of potential welfare compromise divided broadly into physical and mental components. Modified from Mellor and Reid (1994) and Mellor (2004).

Compromise to welfare within these five domains may be illustrated thus.

- *Nutritional* compromise may result from inadequate fluid or food intake or from dietary nutrient imbalances (deficiency or excess), which in turn may lead to greater than normal thirst or hunger, or to feelings of weakness or debility.
- Compromise in the *environmental* domain may be due to outdoor exposure to extreme weather (cold or hot) or, indoors, to uncomfortable or injurious floors or other physical structures, and these may lead, respectively, to hypothermic or hyperthermic distress or to persistent discomfort or pain from bruises, joint problems, skin irritation and so on.
- Compromised *health* may occur in response to traumatic injury, disease agents or toxins, genetic disorders or other forms of functional impairment, and these may lead to a wide range of unpleasant experiences including breathlessness, nausea, sickness, pain, distress, fear or anxiety.
- *Behavioural* compromise may result from severe space restrictions, or over-crowding and agonistic interactions. There may be a lack of substrates allowing the expression of species-specific motivation to perform behaviour patterns such as foraging/hunting, play and exploration, developing a safe resting area, normal mating or parenting behaviour, and positive social interaction, or a general lack of productive occupation, stimulation and opportunity for performing actions with satisfying consequences. Outcomes in terms of mental experience may include anxiety, fear, frustration, helplessness, loneliness and boredom.
- Compromise in the *mental* domain arises from sensory and other neural inputs linked to compromise in the four largely physical or functional domains (nutritional, environmental, health, behavioural), together with cognitive-neural inputs and activity related to external challenge (e.g. situations eliciting 'fight' or 'flight' responses), which are all integrated and expressed mentally as varying degrees of thirst, hunger, weakness, debility, breathlessness, nausea, sickness, pain, distress, fear, anxiety, helplessness, boredom and so on.

Clearly, the greater the intensity of these negative subjective experiences or feelings (in the mental domain), the greater is the associated compromise to an animal's welfare. Although it is not clear how the relative noxiousness of these different experiences may be compared, it is likely that any associated suffering increases as the negative intensity of each rises towards its maximum (see Chapter 5).

1.5 Good Animal Welfare is more than the Mere Absence of Negative Experiences

Minimizing or avoiding such welfare compromises would obviously be beneficial for animals, but the mere absence of such negative experiences cannot necessarily be taken to represent *good* welfare. Nevertheless, a 'neutral' state might be regarded as *acceptable* welfare and could be a considerable improvement in some circumstances. Also, the minimization or avoidance of negative feelings such as those listed above may free the animal to have some positive experiences without further intervention.

A view that is gaining ground is that good welfare probably also depends on the presence of positive experiences or feelings as well as the absence of negative ones (Duncan, 1996; Fraser and Duncan, 1998; Yeates and Main, 2008), and this may require additional interventions. It follows from this view that other forms of animal welfare compromise may arise from an absence of positive mental states related to absence of feelings of reward or satisfaction. Such compromise may therefore occur in circumstances which hinder an animal's capacity to experience, for instance vitality, companionship, contentment, satiety, happiness, curiosity, exploration, foraging and play (Fraser and Duncan, 1998).

The notion that a good state of welfare exists when the nutritional, environmental, health, behavioural and mental needs of an animal are met accommodates all of these considerations. That is because meeting the mental needs of animals can be taken to incorporate both the absence of demonstrably negative experiences and the presence of positive experiences that are shown to be important to the animal.

1.6 Synopsis: A Needs-Based View Integrates Several Key Features of Animal Welfare

Based on the considerations outlined above, it is now possible to characterize animal welfare using a needs-based orientation. A good state of welfare may be said to exist when the nutritional, environmental, health, behavioural and mental needs of conscious higher (sentient) animals are met. This occurs when negative states are absent and/or positive states are present. The five areas of need represent domains of potential welfare compromise, the first four being largely physical or functional, and the last, mental state, representing cognitive and affective attributes of the animal's experience. Thus, sensory and other neural inputs associated with the nutritional, environmental, health and behavioural domains, together with additional cognitive inputs, are processed and then express themselves within the mental domain in terms of the animal's conscious subjective experience. In other words, the welfare status of an animal, whether good, neutral or bad, represents the integrated outcome of all sensory and other neural inputs from within its body and from the environment, inputs which are processed and interpreted by the animal's brain according to its species-specific and individual nature and experience, and then perceived consciously.

1.7 Animal Welfare can be 'Assessed' but not 'Measured'

Although the notion of scoring a particular aspect of the welfare of an animal or group of animals (e.g. pain status) may be attractive in some respects

(Scott *et al.*, 2003), no single, specific or decisive measurement of *overall* animal welfare status has yet emerged, and nor is that likely. This is because such a notion is too simplistic. As indicated above, an animal's welfare status reflects its internal subjective experience, and this represents the integrated outcome of numerous inputs to the animal's brain that result in a wide range of positive, neutral or negative experiences or feelings, none of which can be measured directly. Moreover, each such experience differs in character. For instance, with regard to negative experiences, thirst is not the same as pain, hunger is different from boredom, breathlessness and nausea differ, and frustration is not the same as any of these. Thus, deriving a single number from a composite of several such attributes of welfare that have previously been scored numerically using indirect indices implies a greater understanding of the attributes themselves, and of relationships between them, than is possible now and is likely in the foreseeable future. Assessment of welfare status requires the exercise of scientifically informed good judgement (see below) supported by comprehensive and careful evaluations of those factors that contribute to an animal's internal subjective experiences. Reference to the five domains of welfare and grading non-numerically the extent of compromise an animal may experience in each of them (Mellor and Reid, 1994; Chapter 5) has been used to effectively support such judgements in the context of the impact of experimental procedures on animals.

1.8 Science is the Vehicle for Revealing Animals' Needs

The generalizations above help to characterize animal welfare in terms of animals' needs. The vehicle for revealing what those needs are and how they can be met is science, allied to rigorous and critical practical field observations (e.g. Kirkwood *et al.*, 2001, 2004).

Nutritional, environmental, production and veterinary sciences have contributed hugely to animal welfare during the last 50 years by defining functional responses and the corrective management of animals faced with, for example, nutrient deficiency or excess, thermal challenge, pathogenic microorganisms, injury and the metabolic demands of high productivity (Mellor and Bayvel, 2008; Chapters 2 and 3). Such production-orientated research improved animal welfare because of the close links between animal health and welfare. However, during the last 20–25 years there has been, in addition, a progressive increase in research with an explicit animal welfare focus. This occurred at least partly because the earlier advances in our understanding of nutrition, environmental impacts and disease allowed research attention to be redirected towards the assessment and management of the behavioural and mental needs of animals (Mellor and Bayvel, 2004, 2008). This same period saw the birth of the new discipline area of animal welfare science; that is, the science concerned with the acquisition and application of the knowledge required to characterize, maintain, restore and promote animal welfare. It currently depends heavily on contributions from disciplines including animal behaviour science and cognitive-neural sciences in particular, but also animal husbandry, biochemistry, genetics, immunology, nutrition, physiology, pharmacology, veterinary pathology and veterinary clinical sciences, as we shall see.

1.9 Science and Good Practice are both needed to Advance Animal Welfare Practically

Advances in welfare management are based on scientific knowledge applied, where necessary, to improve currently accepted 'good practice', and on existing good practice that has been validated scientifically. Good practice may be characterized thus (Mellor, 2004b):

- it represents a standard of care that has a wide level of acceptance among knowledgeable practitioners and experts in the field;
- it is based on good sense and sound judgement;
- it is practical and thorough;
- it has robust experiential or scientific foundations;
- it prevents unreasonable or unnecessary harm to, or promotes the interests of, the animals to which it is applied.

Good practice therefore highlights the importance of direct experience with the practical care and management of animals in the circumstances of their use, as well as common sense which has been carefully evaluated. It also depends on knowledgeable observation of animals' health and welfare status, veterinary medicine, and the use of available technology. Scientific knowledge alone is not enough; it must be allied to sound practical experience.

1.10 All Systems for Managing Animals have Positive and Negative Attributes, and Evolve

Systems used to manage animals are retained because they largely meet the purposes for which they were originally devised and because those purposes are judged at the time to be generally acceptable. Positive attributes of commercial farming systems include, for example, high levels of animal productivity, health and, during the last 20 years, welfare, and must also include economic viability (McInerney, 1998; Mellor and Stafford, 2001). Likewise, the beneficial purposes of keeping pet, recreational and sports animals relate to an evident human desire for, among other things, animal-based companionship and nurturing, leisure pursuits and competition (Chapter 7).

However, all such systems have some negative impacts. In farm animals, requiring high productivity may lead to metabolic 'burnout' (e.g. high-yielding dairy cows, end-of-lay or 'spent' hens), space restrictions may hinder normal behavioural expression or produce aberrations (e.g. layer-hen cages, sow stalls), infectious disease problems may be greater in animals kept indoors on deep litter (e.g. indoor lambing), distressing or fatal exposure to weather extremes may be greater outdoors (e.g. pastorally farmed animals) and so on. Examples in other animals include leaving pet dogs (pack animals) alone at home for much of each day, grossly overfeeding or otherwise mismanaging the diet of pet dogs or cats, keeping flocking pet birds alone in extremely small cages, keeping recreational horses in isolation from others, exposing competition horses to a high likelihood of severe injury (e.g. during show jumping, eventing and racing) and so on.

Despite such negative impacts, no system is static. Over time, systems may be modified in an attempt to reduce their detrimental effects on the animals, or new systems may be created to replace ones with apparently intractable problems (Chapters 2 and 3). Further drivers for change are increases in scientific under-standing about the nature of animals' needs, how those needs can be met, and on that basis what are then regarded as acceptable and unacceptable ways of managing animals (Chapters 7 and 8). Moreover, public interest in, and concern about, how animals are managed in specific circumstances (e.g. layer hens in cages, sows in stalls), with input from animal advocate organizations, also influences the approach of animal users, professional advisors (including veterinarians) and regulators (Mellor and Bayvel, 2004, 2008; Chapter 9).

All of these drivers have led to changes in the management systems for farm animals during the last 50 years, and especially the last 25 years (Chapters 2–4). Although the focus for change was always improvement (however judged), unforeseen negative consequences sometimes arose. For instance, improving the then poor hygiene, nutritional management, health and productivity of free-range layer hens by introducing the first cages led, among other things, to the foot or bone problems and the overcrowding and behavioural restrictions which are now of concern. Likewise, use of sow stalls to more efficiently and effectively manage nutrition, hygiene, health and aggression-induced injuries, and to improve productivity, led to leg and back problems, vaginal-vulval inflammation, contact-rubbing injuries or behavioural anomalies (including stereotypies) in a significant proportion of animals.

In terms of animal welfare, therefore, most systems for managing animals have strengths (i.e. the welfare benefits) and weaknesses (i.e. the welfare compromises of different types that may occur), but they also have safeguards. These safeguards are the recommended minimum standards in codes of practice which are directed both at minimizing particular compromises and at promoting positive welfare. Although consideration of all three features (strengths, weaknesses, safeguards) is required when deciding whether or not the *net* welfare status of animals in different systems will be acceptable, the extent to which the safeguards are successfully implemented is clearly of major importance.

1.11 Animal Welfare Trade-Offs should be Managed Responsibly and Re-Assessed Regularly

Many current problems can now be seen as issues that have been 'over-solved'. For instance, the layer hen completely removed from contact with faeces is entirely protected from disease vectors found within them with 100% success: in those terms. Taking a wider view, however, it is evident that no animal is ever really 100% protected. Trade-offs *must* be made, often in broad terms, between the human-centred purpose of using the animal and the animal's own needs, as well as trade-offs between the animal's safety and its freedom. The more opportunities and choices an animal has the more injuries and suffering it may experience if it is unlucky or if those responsible for it are not fully conscientious in their care and monitoring.

We, all of us, decide how to balance these various considerations even as we try to make improvements in all of the domains of welfare and the overall success of the animal, as well as any associated industry and community. To achieve this we not only need agreement between observers within our immediate discipline but between a wider group representing other disciplines and allied professions, and in our wider society (providing social licence). We need to satisfy, as best we can but inevitably not fully, a range of diverse economic, social and ethical imperatives (Fisher and Mellor, 2008).

The discipline of animal welfare science requires as a fundamental quality what could be summed up by the old latin motto of *circumspice*, i.e. 'look around'. This book is an attempt to highlight the need for all of us in the animal welfare arena to constantly *look around* in order to appreciate what we are doing, where we have made progress, and not only when we fail but *whom* we fail, how we fail them and whether what we are doing is really the best that we can do. If we must make trade-offs with an animal's care, it behoves us to do so openly, ethically and mindfully.

Part 2

Paths from the Past

Agricultural Sciences and Animal Welfare

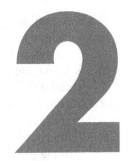

Crop Production and Animal Production

2.1 Some Historical Perspectives

2.1.1 Human lifestyles, population growth and changes in agricultural practices are closely linked

The human requirement for food, of plant and animal origin, has increased as the human population has increased. In the past, the constraints placed on food availability by dependence on gathering, scavenging and hunting was a major factor that limited the human population to around 4 million people (Tilman *et al.*, 2002). The domestication of plants, the advent of agriculture and the later domestication of livestock species and poultry greatly increased the quantities of food available for human consumption with the result that the earth can now feed 6 billion people.

In Eurasia, the use of cattle and buffalo, and later horses, as draught animals to cultivate grain crops such as barley, wheat and rice, increased productivity. This allowed a shift from subsistence to commercial agriculture, which enabled more people to live away from the land. In the Americas, the domestication of maize, squash, beans and potatoes supported the civilizations of Central America (Maya, Aztec) and South America (Inca). Thus, the domestication of crops, followed by livestock and poultry, changed human lifestyles from hunter–gatherer to sedentary subsistence modes and, thereafter, the advent of commercial farming supported urbanization and later industrialization (Diamond, 2002).

It is evident that these substantial improvements in agricultural productivity have sustained the huge growth in the human population, especially over the last century (Trewavas, 2002). As a result, famines are now usually a direct result of warfare or severe climatic conditions (usually drought), and today poor distribution of food contributes more than global underproduction to ongoing problems of starvation and malnutrition. Indeed, efficient production of food, its ready availability (in many countries) and its relatively low cost have now resulted in obesity becoming as great a problem for human health as starvation (Shaw, 2007). Nevertheless, global climate change may be anticipated to increase the likelihood of famine in some areas of the world.

2.1.2 Agricultural development was slow before the advent of agricultural science

Changes in agriculture were relatively slow until the nineteenth century when agriculture became a subject for scientific enquiry; this enhanced basic knowledge of soil types, fertilizer use and crop rotation as well as plant and animal breeding. The twentieth century saw major developments in crop production and thereafter livestock and poultry production, particularly after 1945 (Martin, 2000).

Agricultural science originally focused on crop and livestock production. In the 1950s, the livestock husbandry and production elements of agricultural science were renamed as 'animal science', and this generic science was then subdivided to reflect increasingly detailed knowledge of its various aspects; subdivisions which have been retained to this day. These include nutrition, housing, reproduction, lactation, growth, meat and fibre production, genetics and veterinary science. Crop production, particularly the production of forages and feed grains, became an important component of livestock and poultry nutrition. Crop production was supported by soil and fertilizer science, knowledge of pesticides and weed control, and improved mechanization. All of these elements, by providing the foundations for knowledgeable agricultural management and control, have had significant impacts on the productivity and welfare of livestock and poultry, and have influenced the welfare of sport and companion animals as well.

2.1.3 A conflict between affordable food and increasing demand may endanger animal welfare

Although the future is uncertain, the human population will probably continue to increase until at least 2050 and with it demand for food (Conklin and Stilwell, 2007). Science is therefore likely to be directed at improving livestock and poultry productivity to meet at least part of this rising demand for food. It is also likely to be directed at minimizing detrimental impacts of this increased demand and of likely climate change on crop- and livestock-production systems. Minimizing adverse effects of evolving economic constraints on animal welfare will also require scientific input.

Economically, the drive to increase agricultural productivity and profitability and to maintain low farm-gate prices conflicts with farmers having the resources to give individual animals appropriate care. These economic drivers generally lead to larger farm sizes and greater use of controlled and confined conditions. Although this may jeopardize the care of individual animals in some cases it may also make it more economical to direct smart technologies at maintaining better health and welfare. Historically, many agricultural animals had greater freedom of movement but it is easy to forget that this was associated with routine suffering and mortality associated with malnutrition, starvation, extreme climates, disease, injury and predation, and carrying out procedures such as slaughter without effective prior stunning.

Agricultural subsidization, particularly in Western Europe, may allow the adoption of uneconomical farm management practices that allow greater behavioural freedom. However, whether or not subsidies are provided, the ongoing unwillingness of the major wholesalers and retailers of livestock products to pay more at the farm gate makes the drive for improved attention to individual animals and improved welfare difficult. In addition, animal feed prices are likely to increase because of a developing conflict between the use of grain for human or animal nutrition while global grain production per person decreases, and the recent drive to use grain, especially maize, for biofuel in the face of dwindling fuel-oil resources can only exacerbate this. Climate change will also impact on this conflict.

2.1.4 Agricultural science improved animal welfare, but the extent of this is often not acknowledged

The changes in agriculture led by science, especially during the last century, have had both good and bad effects on animal welfare. In the recent past, many of the benefits for animals have not been acknowledged because of a strong focus on the welfare problems that arose with intensified and industrialized systems during the period before animal welfare science emerged as a research area. Nevertheless, when compared with the pre-scientific period, there have been marked overall improvements in the quality of life of farm animals throughout the period of the application of science to agriculture.

The overall animal welfare benefits of agricultural science arose through advances in soil science, fertilizer utilization and crop production, as well as pasture management, harvesting and storage, together with animal nutrition, environmental regulation and slaughter. The contributions of agricultural science to animal welfare have therefore arisen through improvements in understanding of crop and animal production, both of which are dealt with in more detail below.

2.2 Crop Production

2.2.1 Management of soil fertility and other features greatly improved agricultural productivity

Soil fertility was maintained historically by farmyard manure and crop rotation. The development of soil science led to the classification of soil types, the development of soil testing and identification of the need to provide lime and other minerals, especially phosphorus, potassium and minor/trace elements. Chemical fertilizers, especially nitrogen, phosphorus and potassium, were essential for the expansion of agricultural productivity in the twentieth century. In the UK, for instance, the amount of nitrogen, phosphorus and potassium applied to grassland increased by 40, 25 and four times, respectively, from 1943 to 1998 (Martin, 2000). Also, the controlled use of urea and nitrogen has allowed the rapid growth of some forage crops. The increase in fertilizer use was perhaps the single most important factor that enhanced overall agricultural productivity during the last half of the twentieth century. Large increases in crop production made available more and more fodder and feedstuffs for animals and poultry and therefore greatly enhanced productivity and contributed to improved welfare in those sectors.

Soil science also identified trace-element deficiencies and excesses which could then be corrected to improve both crop production and animal health. For example, in New Zealand cobalt deficiency was identified in the 1930s as a major limitation to cattle and sheep production in the central North Island (Ellison, 2002). Once recognized, cobalt supplementation of soil to improve cobalt levels in forage and/or direct cobalt or vitamin B_{12} dosing of animals allowed healthy growth of lambs and cattle (see below). Similarly, when soils with excess selenium were identified in North America, Ireland and other areas worldwide, preventative measures could be put in place to protect cattle and horses against selenium toxicity. This allowed the successful free-range use of high-production livestock on arable land worldwide and improved the vigour and welfare of animals kept in both old and new pasturelands.

2.2.2 Crop breeding increased the vigour, range and disease resistance of agricultural plants

The science of crop breeding allowed the development of new, more productive breeds of plants which are more resistant to pests and disease. In the UK, it is estimated that nearly half of the increase in crop and grassland productivity since 1945 was due to plant breeding (Martin, 2000). Short-straw wheat and winter-resistant barley made grain production easier, and yield per hectare increased substantially. The breeding of grasses with improved leaf-to-stem ratios and winter tolerance increased grass production. Ryegrass cultivars with low endophyte (e.g. fungus) levels reduced problems with toxicity (e.g. facial eczema) (Smith and Towers, 2002). Also, specialist forage crops of many types (brassicas, silage maize, oats, feeding barley, etc.) were developed. All of these developments helped to improve the range, overall supply and out-of-season availability of forages and feedstuffs and thereby contributed to reductions in animal welfare compromise in the nutritional domain.

Agronomists and animal scientists continue to seek new forage plants with agronomic characteristics that are suited to different environments and for feeding different animal species under different conditions. Traditional breeding selection technology and genetic engineering will continue to produce cultivars of forage crops that are more productive and easier to grow.

2.2.3 Fungicide, pesticide and herbicide development greatly increased plant productivity

The development of plant pathology with the concomitant ability to identify, prevent and treat plant diseases has had a significant effect on our ability to produce food for people and animals. The production of fungicides and pesticides to treat plant diseases and herbicides to control weeds allowed for more controlled production of forage and grain crops. In 1944, there were 65 approved pesticides in the UK, but in 1980 there were 800 (Martin, 2000). These allow for quite specific application of chemicals to kill specific pests.

A major factor in preventing crops reaching their potential was weed competition. The development of herbicides to control broadleaf weeds in crops and weed-specific herbicides allowed greater crop yield, grass production and easier harvesting. Improved grain production in particular has supported the intensive poultry-, pig- and cattle-production systems that developed during the last 40 years and had some health and welfare benefits.

2.2.4 Improved pasture-management, irrigation and farm systems have been important

A major development in pasture utilization arose from improvements in pasture management. The development of electric fences allowed controlled access to feed and gave more control over and more effective use of forage crops and grasses. Rotational grazing replaced set-stocking under specific conditions, particularly in the temperate dairy grasslands of countries such as New Zealand and Ireland (Holmes *et al.*, 2002). This allowed better control of grass utilization and helped to ensure grass would be available for livestock during periods of scarcity – such as in winter – with clear health and welfare benefits.

People have little control over weather, but irrigation allows some control over water supply to plants, and weather forecasting allows for some prediction of when to plant and harvest. The development of irrigation systems increased the areas available for crop and forage production for human, livestock and poultry consumption. They have also protected livestock, particularly dairy cows, from the danger of drought and low rainfall. Water reticulation, drainage and development of cheap farm road systems and vehicles (e.g. all-terrain vehicles) have all made the management of extensively farmed sheep and cattle herds easier. All of these developments have improved the welfare of stock farmed extensively.

2.2.5 Agricultural engineering improved arable land productivity and animal welfare

Developments in agricultural engineering have had significant effects on crop production and directly and indirectly on animal welfare. Until the twentieth century crop production worldwide was dependent on animal traction and the physical effort of people. In temperate climates, traditional animal farming practices relied on the production of forages and grain, usually hay, for feeding ruminants and equids during the winter, and in the tropics feed needed to be conserved for dry- or wet-season feeding. The development of steam power and the combustion engine in the nineteenth century made crop production easier. The mechanization of agriculture became widespread in the twentieth century and allowed farms to become larger and more efficient. For instance, in 1939 horses were doing more than two-thirds of the work on farms in the UK. In 1945, there were 436 000 working horses in England and Wales, whereas in 1965 there were only 20 000

(Martin, 2000). Using horses for work is now exceptionally rare. The feeding of draft horses was a major limitation for peasant and smaller farms as food, including grain, had to be grown for the horse even when it was not working.

Horse and cattle power limited the development of extensive commercial agriculture, whereas mechanization supported it by allowing efficient use of optimal ploughing, seeding and harvesting times (Martin, 2000). For example, the development of the combine harvester, which could harvest grain directly, without the need for separate cutting and threshing, allowed more efficient use of often limited suitable weather and allowed the cropping of large areas by fewer people. Development of machinery also facilitated more efficient use of fertilizer and pesticides via topdressing using tractors or aircraft. Moreover, the development of mowers, turners, rakes and balers made hay production safer, and more recent mechanization led to more efficient production of silage and haylage. All of these are easier to produce than the traditional winter livestock feed crop, hay, and can be made during shorter periods and are therefore less weather-dependent. Mechanization also facilitated the production of forage crops such as turnips, kale and rape for feeding animals during times of grass shortage such as in winter, thereby helping to avoid seasonal starvation of livestock such as dairy cattle, which occurred commonly and was severe in many regions.

In the developed world, mechanization ended the use of horses and bullocks for road, farm and military work, and an associated reduction in their numbers had a major impact on their welfare. For instance, horses were often worked in appalling conditions and mechanization ended this more effectively than did any legislation. In developing countries, working animals are common (Figure 2.1)

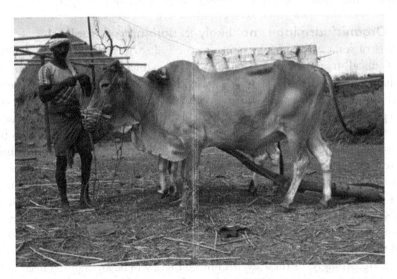

Figure 2.1 Draught Zebu bullocks in the Yemen (©2009, K.J. Stafford, reproduced with permission).

Table 2.1 Changes in human and animal populations and wheat production during the last five decades (Food and Agriculture Organisation databases).

| Year | Populations (billions) | | | | Wheat production (million tonnes) |
	Human	Cattle	Pigs	Chickens	
1961	2.6	0.9	0.4	3.9	222
1970	3.6	1.1	0.5	5.2	310
1980	4.4	1.2	0.8	7.2	440
1990	5.2	1.3	0.9	10.7	592
2000	6.0	1.3	0.9	14.5	586
2006	6.5	1.4	1.0	16.9	605

and their condition can be deplorable. Animal traction (e.g. horse, donkey, mule, bullock, camel, elephant) still provides the greater element of power in farming in many parts of Africa and Asia, and the welfare of these animals is often poor, particularly during the ploughing and planting seasons and when used for threshing grains. Replacement of traction animals with mechanical alternatives is expensive, and this will limit their adoption in less affluent regions.

Developments in the mechanics of harvesting, drying and storage of grain crops have made this a safer and more controlled activity, and allowed for grain surplus to human need to be used for stock and poultry feed (Table 2.1). Such developments have also increased the production of food specifically destined for livestock and poultry and made it safer, less weather-dependent and cheaper.

2.2.6 'Organic' farming is not likely to dominate globally

The desire of some advocates to return to pre-industrial agricultural methodology with 'chemical'-free agricultural techniques ('organic' farming) is unlikely to be more than a luxury affordable only in wealthier regions of the world. Chemical-free agriculture will not meet the requirement for food by the human population, expected to reach 9 billion by 2050. Indeed, the world's demand for food is expected to double by 2050 (Green *et al.*, 2005). If this population is to be fed using organic farming systems then more land will be needed than is under agricultural production at present. Most of the best agricultural land is already under cultivation (Tilman *et al.*, 2002). Moreover, low-chemical farming is likely to impede farmers' abilities to produce food for livestock under controlled circumstances. This is significant because livestock and poultry production will almost certainly contribute to meeting the rising need for food. For instance, the efficiency of poultry and pig systems will probably ensure that egg and white-meat production will continue. Accordingly, as these events unfold there will be an ongoing need to manage the consequences of 'organic' practices for animal welfare, and animal-based sciences will play a major part in that. However, the commitment of the 'organic' movement to managing livestock with no or low-chemical inputs may have some beneficial outcomes if it reveals and properly validates approaches that maintain productivity and welfare with much reduced chemical use or effective alternative inputs or management strategies (see Chapter 3).

2.3 Animal Production and Animal Welfare

Scientific interest in livestock and poultry production dates back at least to the nineteenth century, but most major developments in our scientific understanding of animal production occurred last century. An emphasis on a scientific basis to production led to a change in university and college departmental names from animal husbandry to animal science. It might also have contributed to a decline in the caring aspect of livestock management – that is, classical husbandry – a trend which may have been reinforced by numerous examples of successful knowledge-based manipulation and control of animal productivity focused on biological health and safety through confinement, rather than on behavioural management.

We have already noted that the key subdivisions of animal science include housing (environments), nutrition, reproduction, lactation, growth, meat and fibre production, genetics and veterinary science. Impacts of veterinary science and genetics on animal welfare will be considered in Chapters 3 and 4, respectively, and aspects of the other areas of science are outlined below using specific examples.

2.3.1 Increased knowledge improved facilities and environments for animals managed indoors and outdoors

In cold climates, some species of livestock such as cattle were traditionally housed during winter but may have been kept outdoors during late spring, summer and autumn. Likewise, pigs and poultry were traditionally managed extensively during summer and housed during winter, but some species like sheep were often kept outdoors at all times.

2.3.1.1 Wintering of cattle indoors

When kept outdoors in temperate climates during winter, cattle can have detrimental effects on pasture production through pugging and sward damage. The development of commercial industrial farming in the temperate latitudes led to cattle being over-wintered indoors. They were often tethered in stalls and held in one place throughout the winter. This is still common in many European countries, especially on farms with small numbers of cattle, because loose housing for cattle is costly. Also, bedding for tethered cows can be used frugally, thereby reducing costs, which contrasts with the more expensive use of bedding for cattle that are loose-housed. Manure management is an important issue with housed cattle, and other stock, and the development of slatted floor sheds in the 1960s, where the faeces fall through the slats into underfloor containment areas, allowed the loose-housing of cattle to be more attractive to producers.

Although loose-housing is a better option than tethering because it allows cattle to move around while held indoors, it has now been found that the cattle themselves prefer to be outdoors on pine bark pads rather than indoors on slatted floors (Hickey *et al.*, 2002).

2.3.1.2 Milking parlour design

Primitive milking parlours and hand milking are common in many parts of the developing world. The development of modern dairy parlours – with milking machines, automated mastitis identification and a design that encourages the free movement of cows into the parlour – has made the milking of cows much easier for people and perhaps less stressful for the cows. The design of dairy parlours has gone through several stages from tie-up and move-through designs, to herringbone and, more recently, rotary designs (Figure 2.2). All of these changes have been made to increase the speed of milking and facilitate cow throughput and human access to the udder (Holmes *et al.*, 2002). In making it easier to milk more cows, these developments facilitated management of larger herds. Whether the welfare of cows is better in small or larger herds is open to debate. Although large-herd owners can afford facilities that owners of smaller herds cannot, they have less time available to give the cows individual attention.

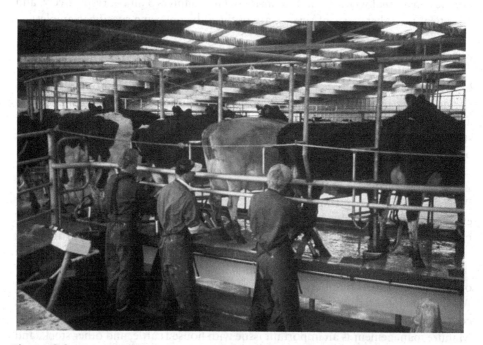

Figure 2.2 Rotary milking parlour (©2009, M.W. Fisher, reproduced with permission).

2.3.1.3 Poultry housing

In the twentieth century, a major revolution in poultry production occurred with a great increase in the housing of layer hens and broiler chickens, and then the caging of layers. This movement indoors depended on and produced improvements in nutrition, disease control and housing. Electricity allowed control of photoperiod and increases to the day length in winter, which enabled egg production to continue past the normal season (Appleby et al., 2004). While this has markedly increased egg production per bird and virtually eliminated parasites and faecal-borne diseases such as coccidiosis, the increased metabolic demands on each bird may have had negative welfare effects. By the 1950s a condition called caged layer fatigue was recognized. This is now understood to result primarily from osteoporosis, and remains a problem in high-producing hens, exacerbated by lack of opportunities for exercise, which further weakens bones (Webster, 2004).

Developments in poultry housing have led to extensive automation so that modern facilities now have automated monitoring and control of air quality, lighting and overall feed and water intakes. Thus, automation, with suitable backup facilities in case of breakdowns, applied to houses containing layer hens in cages and broiler chickens in loose housing, provides for all of the physical needs of the birds and as such has helped to maintain their physical well-being (Figure 2.3). Efficient rodent control is another major advantage of intensive indoor poultry-production systems. As noted in Chapter 1, when instituted these developments improved the health, hygiene and welfare of the birds from their previous state, but they now raise welfare concerns related to barren environments, overcrowding and behavioural restrictions. Thus, developments aiming to protect have ultimately restricted locomotion and behaviour in what might be considered an over-correction.

In contrast, the management of hens outdoors does not allow the same level of control of their environment. Flock sizes are usually smaller with outdoor than indoor systems. Food wastage may be greater and disease control, particularly parasite control, is not as easy outdoors. Physical discomfort and predation are important welfare issues, and management of chickens outdoors requires greater labour inputs than does their management indoors, with great variation in both animal welfare and food safety. Currently, public opinion supports a return to providing hens with greater behavioural freedom, but wider recognition is required of the welfare risks to hens in less intensive systems, especially with large commercial flocks where injurious pecking and disease outbreaks can spread rapidly.

2.3.1.4 Pig housing

The management of pigs in countries such as Papua New Guinea and parts of Central America is probably similar to traditional approaches to pig production in Europe. In such systems, pigs are fed waste-food materials, and are allowed to forage. Parasite infestation is common and mortality rates of piglets are high. In Europe, however, pig-management systems have moved from individual sows owned by peasants and country people, through larger herds held in pens and sties

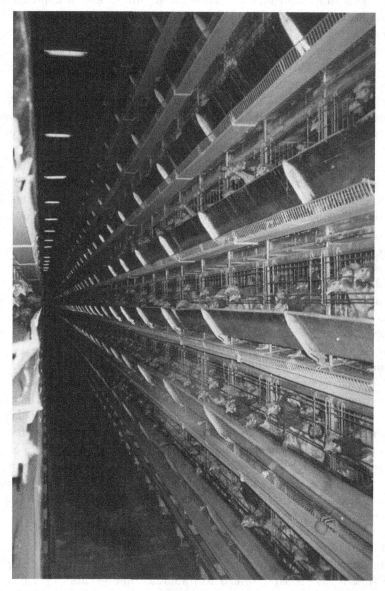

Figure 2.3 Cage housing for layer hens (©2009, M.W. Fisher, reproduced with permission).

and often allowed to forage, to large pig farms with hundreds of sows and pigs for rearing. During the last 50 years, intensification of the pig industry has paralleled that of the poultry industry. The number of weaners per sow per year has risen in the UK from 12.8 in 1950 to 21.5 in 1995 (Martin, 2000). This was accompanied by increased protection of piglets by farrowing crates developed in the 1950s, and infrared lamps to keep piglets warm. Farrowing crates and safe areas reduced piglet mortality but limited the space available to sows and prevented them from making a farrowing nest. The age of weaning was also decreased from around 8 weeks in the 1960s to less than 5 weeks at present, to allow sows to have more litters per year (Martin, 2000). Although the design of farrowing crates may change to allow sows more movement, the basic concept of allowing piglets to get away from the sows remains important for their safety.

Control of access to food is particularly important in pregnant sows, as they will overeat if allowed. Stalls enabled control of individual food intakes and also reduced aggressive exchanges between sows, but long-term close confinement in stalls remains of key welfare concern. Computer control of food delivery to individual sows now allows food intake to be limited using transponders so that sows can be group-housed without the danger of overeating. Houses for finishing pigs have regulated environments with automated air quality, temperature and lighting control. Maintaining even temperatures allows for a better food-conversion ratio (i.e. mass of food eaten/body mass produced), which has decreased from 4.5 to 2.5 (see Martin, 2000). The welfare problems associated with intensification have resulted in an increase in outdoor sow systems and a return to group-housing on straw in sheds, which was popular in the 1950s.

2.3.1.5 Sheep managed outdoors, lambing managed indoors

Traditionally, sheep were farmed and lambed outdoors, and were provided with limited supplementary feeding. In some countries, it may be cost effective to feed preserved forages and grain to counter lamb losses experienced with outdoor lambing systems, and in temperate climates there is a trend for more ewes to be lambed indoors. Ewes that are used to the presence of humans are not distressed when managed indoors (Fisher and Mellor, 2002). However, where sheep are managed extensively, as in Australia and New Zealand, lambing outdoors is usual.

2.3.1.6 Yard and race design

The design of effective yards and other facilities for handling ruminants was based on the experiences of farmers with large sheep flocks to shear and cattle herds to manage. Many of the designs seen in old yards are still appropriate, but during the last 40 years behavioural scientists have investigated the movement of sheep, cattle and pigs through yards and races of different designs and have recommended adjustments to improve movement. These developments, applied to yards in slaughter plants, have facilitated movement and reduced the stress experienced by animals en route to the stunning pen (see Grandin, 1993).

2.3.2 Nutritional science enhanced productivity-based feeding and overall animal welfare

In the eighteenth and nineteenth centuries, the science of animal nutrition identified carbohydrates, fats and proteins as being necessary nutrients. However, it was not until the last half of the twentieth century that nutritional science flourished and we gained a detailed knowledge of vitamins, amino acids, fatty acids, inorganic elements and the specific nutrient requirements of animals in different physiological states such as pregnancy, lactation and growth (Pond *et al.*, 2004). More than 40 nutrients required in the diets of various species have now been identified, and this list may not yet be complete. Parallel to these advances was an improved ability to manufacture nutrients for inclusion as additives in diets. Our knowledge of digestive physiology, biochemistry and metabolism also has increased greatly during the last 60 years. These advances in the science and technology of nutrition have resulted in improved diet formulations. These enhanced our ability to feed an adequate diet to different species of animals in different physiological states, with obvious benefits to their welfare. Novel solutions to nutrient supply were also sought. However, although greater efficiencies were gained by acquiring feedstuff nutrients from non-traditional sources, unexpected risks sometimes emerged, such as when meat-and-bone meal fed to cattle led to the spread bovine spongiform encephalopathy (so-called mad cow disease).

2.3.3 A combination of factors changed cattle-production systems

In the developed world, cattle-production systems changed greatly in the twentieth century, and there was scientific input into both the initiation of change and assessment of the results. Friesian and Holstein cows became the dominant dairy breeds, and the development of progeny testing and use of artificial insemination facilitated the widespread use of a limited number of bulls with high production potential, but sometimes poor conformation. The number of lactations before culling (longevity) decreased considerably in association with the increased productivity of modern dairy cows. Improvements in forage production and preservation, and increased feeding of grain, provided a more reliable source of feed for cattle, and developments in milking-machine design made the management of larger herds possible. Winter housing using self-feed silage and indoor cubicles made winter management easier. The increase in herd size had both positive and negative effects on welfare; positive, in that large dairy farms can afford the methods and advice to manage cows effectively, but negative in that less attention may be given to the welfare of individual cows. Larger units can afford to train staff, but paid managers may not have the personal investment of farmer owners.

Traditionally, ruminants were fed grass, hay and the straw or stover from cereal crops, and perhaps some grain if they were used for traction. During the last century the feeding of grain to cattle increased, particularly to dairy cattle in Europe and North America and to beef cattle in feedlots in North America. This increase in feeding grain and an associated reduction in intakes of roughage caused health

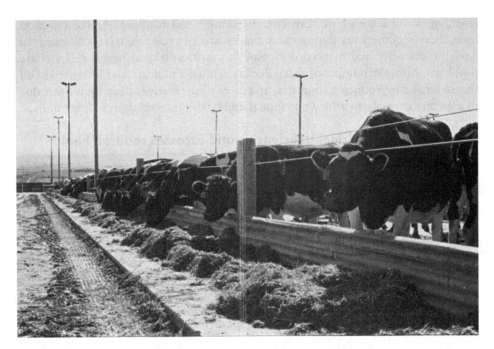

Figure 2.4 Feedlot cattle (©2009, M.W. Fisher, reproduced with permission).

problems which nevertheless can be prevented by improved feeding of roughage (Figure 2.4). Increased productivity by dairy cows such as Holsteins made the feeding of grain essential if they were to meet milk-production targets. However, intensively fed high-producing cows are not retained for long and some may be culled before the end of their second lactation. This suggests that such animals have been pushed beyond what is truly biologically sustainable into a state, described as metabolic burnout, which is inimical to good welfare.

Beef production, particularly finishing, has become more intensive with the development of feedlots and the feeding of grain. Use of feedlots allows close observation of individual cattle and may make it easier to identify, restrain and treat injured or diseased animals. However, transporting weaner calves long distances from calf-rearing farms to feedlots and feeding a grain diet have implications for respiratory and gastric diseases, respectively.

2.3.4 Defining the nutrient requirements of sheep greatly improved their health and welfare

The quantitative determination during the 1960s and 1970s of the nutrient requirements of sheep, especially with regard to energy, protein, minerals and trace elements, enabled their nutrition to be managed knowledgeably throughout their life cycle. The different requirements of pregnant, lactating, growing and mature animals were defined and this information, combined with the concurrently emerging knowledge of the capacity of pasture and available forage crops to meet those requirements during the annual seasonal cycle, led to much-improved lamb productivity and marked decreases in nutrition-related health and welfare problems. Also, the number of sheep flocks declined and flock sizes increased in all the major sheep-producing countries, and there were positive effects on welfare due to a greater capacity to afford nutritional and health interventions in large units.

2.3.5 Managing nutrient deficiencies and excesses reduced health and welfare problems

A further important development in livestock nutrition was the recognition that some soil types are deficient in particular trace elements – notably cobalt, copper, iodine or selenium – which are required if livestock are to remain healthy. In New Zealand, as noted above, recognition in the 1930s that volcanic soils are deficient in cobalt and cause ill-thrift in cattle and sheep (Figure 2.5) led to the supplementation of animals with either cobalt or vitamin B_{12} as a preventative measure. Conversely, some soils have excess trace elements either naturally, for example selenium, or due to industrial contamination, for example copper and fluorine. These cause toxicity-related health and welfare problems which are avoided by not using such land for grazing or by restricting grazing to short periods.

2.3.6 Nutritional science contributed to the industrialization of poultry production

There was a revolution in egg and poultry meat production during the last half of the twentieth century where small production units were replaced by huge factory farms. The recognition that vitamin D could be fed to chickens in cod-liver oil made intensive housing of poultry possible as the birds no longer needed to be exposed

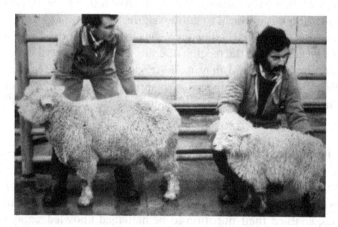

Figure 2.5 Normal (left) and cobalt-deficient (right) lambs (©2009, D. West, reproduced with permission).

to sunlight (Appleby *et al.*, 2004). Compounding feeds for poultry had commenced before this, but as dietary requirements were clarified appropriate supplementation with required minerals and vitamins became possible. The manufacture of synthetic amino acids in the 1950s also made the supplementation of poultry diets easier and cheaper. Diets are now made specifically for the type of poultry, for example high-energy, high-protein diets for broilers. In addition, the improved control of disease, air quality, ambient temperature, photoperiod and brooding, plus automation of feeding and waste removal, allowed flock sizes to grow rapidly. In 1967 in the UK, the average cage-laying flock size was 2200 birds but in 2000, 97% of layers were in flocks of 20 000 or more (Appleby *et al.*, 2004). Likewise, in the broiler industry flock size has increased substantially. The industrialization of poultry production has had positive and negative effects on poultry welfare. Health, hygiene, nutrition, environmental stability and air quality have improved, but the opportunity to behave in anything resembling a normal manner has been prevented by limited space and barren facilities, especially for caged layers.

2.3.7 Improved nutritional management contributed to intensification of pig production

As already noted, pig productivity increased substantially during the last half century with regard to the reproductive efficiency of sows and feed-conversion rates (Martin, 2000). The conflict on the one hand between the intensive systems which have enabled increased production and improved health, nutritional and environmental control, and on the other hand the thwarted needs of pigs to nest and forage, remains in those units that rely on continuous close confinement in sow stalls. The concentration of pig production on fewer farms is similar to that seen in the poultry industry and in other livestock-production systems worldwide.

There is some movement towards outdoor production of piglets and straw-bedded shed systems for growing pigs. The former has some welfare implications regarding piglet mortality. Arks may be dirty and perhaps cold for piglets, and if soils are not free-draining then sow yards may become muddy. Straw-bedded sheds allow growing pigs to engage in a range of behaviours while still being fed efficiently. These may replace slatted floors in areas where straw is cheap and readily available.

2.3.8 Companion animal diets are formulated scientifically and produced industrially

The companion animal food industry is a product of the late twentieth century. Previously, dogs depended on household waste or scraps from the local butchery. The development of a pet-food industry depended on knowledge accrued by nutritionists and the development of manufacturing ability. It is now estimated that at least 70% of dog-owning households in the UK feed their dogs on commercial dog food, and 90% of calories fed to dogs in the USA, Japan and northern Europe are from commercial pet food, but figures are less than 60 and 50% in the UK and France, respectively (see Hand *et al.*, 2000). The situation with cats is likely to be similar. Developments in nutritional science mean that pet food can now be formulated to contain all essential nutrients, with species-specific additives such as taurine in feline diets.

There is currently a movement away from commercial food towards raw-food diets of bones and meat, but claims of long-term health or longevity benefits are unproven. However, such fresh diets, or mixtures of commercial pet food and some meat or bones, may be more 'interesting' to dogs and cats, and are often advocated by veterinarians (Stafford, 2006). In contrast, there are now specialist dog and cat foods designed for animals with particular physiological needs such as rapid growth, pregnancy and aging, and for specific disease problems such as liver or kidney disease and allergies. There are even special diets formulated for over-indulged obese dogs.

2.4 The Future

2.4.1 Past achievements show that further marked improvements in animal health and welfare are likely

Past improvements in the production of food for livestock, housing designs and disease control provide a sound basis for ongoing development in livestock and poultry production systems, and allow concurrent enhancement of animal welfare. Advances made possible by confinement could be refined if the advantages of safe, clean enclosures could be retained while steps are taken to allow more normal behaviours to be performed.

Current welfare debates are often framed as a dichotomy with the negative effects of confinement compared with the traditionally based philosophies of free-range and organic farming (Webster, 1994). As noted above, however, the advances of agricultural science over the last century have largely been beneficial, not only for efficient and safe food production, but also for the overall health and welfare of the animals. Yet, in avoiding disease vectors and the negative effects of aggression, confinement agriculture can be seen as having taken a strategy of containment too far in not allowing animals to exercise and express behaviours.

However, the solution need not be a step back to systems that reintroduce conquered risks of malnutrition and exposure to disease vectors, predation and climatic extremes. Agricultural science contains within it the solutions to its flaws and, given the opportunity, could correct its own excesses. A good example is the way in which food intake by individual animals can be controlled by computer systems which allow animals to range freely, either outdoors or indoors, without loss of control of their food intake. Individual monitoring of behaviour and health of free-ranging animals in extensive systems using smart technologies will also allow rapid identification of sick or injured animals and aid immediate restraint and treatment. Also, global positioning systems will allow farmers to identify where animals are and to manage forages appropriately. It is likely that many of the developments in livestock and poultry production in the next few decades will be constrained or accelerated by welfare requirements.

We must mindfully balance the need to contain the animal and ensure its safety from disease and conspecific aggression with the need to free the animal to exercise its body and satisfy its behavioural motivations. Currently, there is much greater public confidence in tradition as a guide to improving animal welfare, but this may be largely because the major problems of traditional systems have receded from our cultural memory and have been replaced with a bucolic mythology. Also, the worst features of scientifically supported confinement are evident to us every day in the form of highly unpopular and widely publicized use of crates and cages. Yet a fair and balanced appreciation of the role of science and customary practices should recognize that agricultural science has provided solutions to immense blights on animal experience in the form of once widely accepted and, at the time, intractable starvation, malnutrition, painful injury and disease. In a world where large-scale agriculture will be absolutely necessary, science may also be the primary method for resolving the arguably less challenging problem of insufficient behavioural freedom.

Veterinary Science and Animal Welfare

3.1 Introduction

In order to highlight some historical developments in animal care, we have sought to show how aspects of the practice of veterinary medicine and surgery and the related contributions of veterinary science have helped to significantly advance animal welfare. Furthermore, we have given attention to some welfare implications of the burgeoning area of the organic management of livestock to provide additional insights into the role of veterinary input and some of its potential disadvantages.

3.1.1 Modern veterinary care evolved over centuries and has relied increasingly on science

The art of managing illnesses, injuries or other disorders of animals goes back millennia and was presumably part of the process of domestication. As individuals, for example farriers, became more specialized in the preventative and therapeutic services they offered, using practices that were considered to be effective at each time in history, the defined roles of veterinary medicine and surgery began to evolve. These veterinary arts were increasingly recognized as legitimate specialties, and were progressively enhanced over the last two centuries by the rigorous application of scientific methodology, especially during the last 50–100 years. Today, veterinary science embodies the evidence-based knowledge that underpins the practice of veterinary medicine and surgery. It also has relevance to a wide range of other areas including livestock production; biosecurity; veterinary public health issues such as zoonoses, or diseases transmitted to humans from animals; food hygiene; drug residues; environmental impacts of animals, perhaps especially production animals; and wildlife management and conservation. More recently, animal welfare science and applied animal behaviour science have been included among the specified key areas of veterinary interest.

3.1.2 Improved health management has enhanced animal welfare worldwide

As already noted, the health of an animal is one of the five essential domains of its welfare. Thus, all past significant improvements in aspects of health management have enhanced animal welfare. This was perhaps especially so from the beginning of the nineteenth century with regard to improvements in the prevention, control and treatment of infectious diseases. Although the related health and therefore welfare benefits applied to animals on individual farms or in local areas, they also extended to national, continental or even global populations of animals. Additional developments that widened the scope of veterinary treatment options, including those involving surgery, paralleled those that occurred in human medicine during the twentieth century and greatly benefited animals.

3.1.3 Economic drivers have influenced the focus of veterinary attention

On-farm economic pressures have influenced developments in veterinary medicine and surgery as they relate to livestock and poultry because of financial limits imposed on the amount of money spent on treatment. Veterinary attention to farm animals therefore emphasized the prevention of disease and the public health aspects of meat and milk production. This was of particular importance because of the comparative economics of preventing versus treating disease and the production losses that occurred with clinical and subclinical disease. Another factor was the commercial value of the animals involved and the likelihood of them returning to full productivity after treatment.

A dramatic change in companion animal medicine that occurred during the last 30 years also had a significant economic dimension. Although companion animals may be worth little in monetary terms they provide company and are family members rather than economic units. Their emotional significance makes treatment expenses an emotional rather than a business issue. Owners are therefore often prepared to spend more on their treatment. In addition, health insurance for companion animals has financed greater expenditure on their medical and surgical care than on the care of production animals (Stafford, 2006).

3.2 Veterinary Medicine and Surgery

3.2.1 Major epidemics gave impetus to the development of veterinary medicine as a professional area

Veterinary medicine has a long history in China and the Middle East. There are frescos in Egypt, from at least 3000 years ago, of a man calving a cow, and Genghis Khan (AD 1155–1227) probably had farrier veterinarians attending his horses. The word veterinarian was used in English for the first time in the seventeenth century. However, the major epidemics of rinderpest in Europe in the eighteenth century, which killed an estimated 200 million cattle during the 68 years after 1711 (Dunlop and Williams, 1996), clearly demonstrated an urgent need to improve veterinary knowledge. The first veterinary school was established in Lyon (France) in 1762 and was quickly followed by others, for example Turin (Italy) in 1769, Gottingen (Germany) in 1771, Copenhagen (Denmark) in 1773, Skara (Sweden) in 1775, Hanover (Germany) in 1778, Budapest (Hungary) in 1787 and London (England) in 1791. Epidemics continued to stimulate veterinary activity; an estimated 400 000 cattle were killed in Britain by rinderpest in 1866. There was also a desire to manage less devastatingly widespread outbreaks of other infectious disease. Thus, in the eighteenth century veterinarians attempted vaccination, for instance, of horses against strangles using pus from strangles abscesses, and cattle against rinderpest using nasal discharges. The concept of using quarantine and control of animal movement to manage disease was well known in the nineteenth century, and rabies was eliminated from Britain and Ireland in the early twentieth century by controlling dog populations and movement of dogs, and by muzzling.

Many more veterinary schools were established in the twentieth century and the number of veterinarians continues to increase worldwide. The number in the American Veterinary Medical Association increased from 23 623 in 1962 to 50 070 in 2000 (Stafford, 2006), and this doubling of veterinarians probably reflects worldwide trends.

3.2.2 Changes in available technology and a need for cheap food influenced the species focus of veterinary activity

Although veterinarians were interested in all domestic species, the horse occupied much of their professional attention until its replacement by steam, diesel and petrol engines around the mid-twentieth century. This development and, after World War II, an emphasis by European governments on improving the availability of cheap meat and eggs, facilitated by an allocation of additional resources for related research and development, led veterinary practitioners and scientists to concentrate on diseases of livestock and poultry. Major veterinary developments occurred in the 1950s and 1960s in disease prevention and vaccine production. More recently, veterinary medicine has become focused increasingly on companion animal health (Table 3.1) so that fewer practising veterinarians now work with livestock or poultry in affluent countries, although this in not the case in many countries in Africa and Asia. This shift towards companion animals, where it has occurred, was at least partly due to the uptake of biomedical technology, surgical techniques and pharmaceuticals by veterinarians with clients who could afford to pay for more costly professional services.

3.2.3 There is a global trend towards increasing specialization in veterinary practice

General veterinary practice, supported by undergraduate curricula, had a multi-species orientation until at least the 1970s. Indeed, the capacity to provide for the

Table 3.1 Predicted employment of veterinarians in the USA (adapted from Brown and Silverman, 1999).

Employment	Year			
	1997	**2000**	**2005**	**2015**
Companion animal	39 875	41 416	44 667	52 741
Large animal	11 728	11 738	11 951	12 081
Industry	1 962	2 009	2 152	2 431
Total[a]	63 351	64 944	68 620	77 317

[a]Includes employment of veterinarians in areas of the profession other than those listed.

Table 3.2 Specialist areas defined by the Royal College of Veterinary Surgeons.

Species-specialist areas	Other specialist areas
Cattle health and production	Anaesthesia
Deer health and production	Behavioural medicine
Equine gastroenterology	Cardiology
Equine medicine	Dentistry
Equine surgery	Dermatology
Exotic animal medicine	Diagnostic imaging
Feline medicine	Epidemiology
Fish health and production	Neurology
Laboratory animal science	Oncology
Pig medicine	Ophthalmology
Poultry medicine and production	Pathology
Sheep health and production	Public health
Small animal surgery	Reproduction
Zoo and wildlife medicine	

wide range of species of veterinary interest in each country was portrayed as a virtue, a source of professional pride. Times changed, so that during the last three decades veterinary practice has become specialized, and some veterinarians work with only one of three classes of animals, namely companion animals, farm animals or horses. In addition, there are now specialists in a range of medical and surgical areas (Table 3.2). This tendency towards specialization had a major influence on the depth of clinical knowledge, and the orientation of undergraduate curricula, and allowed the development of referral practices with specialists in several subject areas. Specialists undertake further postgraduate training in their area of interest and are usually registered with national registration bodies such as the Royal College of Veterinary Surgeons in the UK, or the Australian College of Veterinary Scientists. Specialties in animal welfare and animal behaviour are now available in Australia and the UK, and are under development in the USA and elsewhere.

3.2.4 Holistic approaches to veterinary practice have increased in recent decades

In contrast to the traditional reactive approach of largely dealing with animal health-related problems as they arose, veterinarians have increasingly adopted a more proactive holistic approach during the last few decades. For instance, practising dairy veterinarians still deal with day-to-day animal health matters such as disease control and treatment, but they now also provide consultancy advice on overall farm-management issues such as economic planning and programming activities to optimize health, production and animal welfare. Likewise, in companion animal practice veterinarians now advise on behaviour, nutrition, genetics and issues such as pet selection, in addition to their more direct day-to-day therapeutic roles. This holistic approach has occurred because the profession recognized that it was needed and because of public demand. Scientifically supported medical and surgical procedures predominate, but some complementary or alternative therapies are also used.

3.3 Veterinary Science

3.3.1 Veterinary science consists of tiered disciplines that underpin the practice of veterinary medicine and surgery

Veterinary science may be envisaged in terms of three tiers, as follows:

- pre-clinical disciplines dealing with *normal function*, which include animal behaviour, anatomy, animal science, biochemistry, histology, pharmacology and physiology;
- para-clinical disciplines dealing with *the causes and nature of health and welfare problems*, which include bacteriology, epidemiology, immunology, parasitology, pathology and virology;
- clinical disciplines dealing with *how to remedy health and welfare problems*, including veterinary medicine and surgery, and their sub-disciplines (Table 3.2).

3.3.2 Major advances in veterinary science have occurred in the last 50–100 years

Successful application of science to veterinary therapeutic practice has been manifest for at least the last 100 years, and especially during the last 50 years. The breadth and depth of developments in all disciplines that underpin veterinary medicine and surgery are evident in the wider content, greater number and increased specialization of published textbooks. For example, in the 1970s there were few textbooks on canine and feline medicine and surgery whereas now there are many. In parallel with this trend, the number and specialization of veterinary science journals also increased.

Numerous early advances in veterinary disciplines relied on developments in the human biomedical arena, but for many decades now research with an animal-specific orientation has been the predominant influence (Mellor and Bayvel, 2008), although animal-based research for human benefit has continued to contribute. Overall, the outcome has been marked improvements in animal disease prevention, diagnosis and treatment, and associated reductions in animal suffering. Veterinary surgery has also advanced greatly. Some of the major veterinary therapeutic advances include sulphonamides and antibiotics to help control infections, anthelmintics for parasite control, anaesthesia (general and local) for pain-free surgery, analgesics including anti-inflammatory agents for longer-lasting pain relief, diuretics to help control some consequences of heart dysfunction and a wide range of vaccines to prevent painful and distressing infectious diseases. The development of vaccines for more than 60 infectious diseases of animals (Table 3.3), even considered alone, is an astounding achievement. All of these developments, and many more including improved understanding of hereditary diseases and their prevention and treatment by gene therapy (see Chapter 4), have occurred through the systematic and painstaking construction of the comprehensive edifice that has become veterinary science.

3.3.3 The huge continuing contribution of veterinary science to reducing animal suffering worldwide is greatly underestimated

It is evident that veterinary scientific activity has been, and continues to be, successfully deployed across species to markedly improve the health and therefore the welfare of many millions of animals. The extent of the associated improvements over the past 50–100 years is greatly underestimated at the present time because of lack of familiarity with how devastating some of the previous health problems were before the intervention of scientifically supported veterinary treatments. The absence of, or the rapid diagnosis and treatment of, these ill-health conditions today also leads to an underestimation of the ongoing benefits of what are now routine veterinary interventions, for example vaccination. Below, we have listed just some of these developments in a small number of species. This is not intended to be a comprehensive account; it is illustrative.

3.3.3.1 Cattle
Infectious diseases
Five major infectious diseases of cattle are rinderpest, contagious bovine pleuro-pneumonia, foot-and-mouth disease (FMD), bovine tuberculosis and brucellosis. They were widespread until focused veterinary scientific activity in the twentieth century led to effective control programmes being developed. They caused suffering and death in a large proportion of affected animals and were also major causes of human distress. Outbreaks now generally occur in countries without effective

Table 3.3   List of infectious disease of animals against which more than 60 vaccines have been developed.

Species	Disease	Species	Disease
Cattle	Anthrax	Sheep	Bluetongue
	Bovine virus diarrhoea		*Campylobacter* abortion
	Brucellosis		Caseous lymphadenitis
	Clostridial diseases		*Chlamydia* abortion
	Contagious bovine pleuropneumonia		Clostridial diseases (>6)
	Foot-and-mouth disease		Contagious pustular dermatitis
	Infectious rhinotracheitis		Foot-and-mouth disease
	Louping-ill		Footrot
	Parasitic lung infections		Johne's disease
	Pasteurellosis		Louping-ill
	Rabies		Pasteurellosis
	Rinderpest		Peste des petits ruminants
	Tuberculosis		Scabby mouth
Pigs	Atrophic rhinitis		Sheep pox
	Aujeszky's disease		*Toxoplasma* abortion
	Coliform enteritis	Poultry	Avian encephalomyelitis
	Hog cholera		Egg drop syndrome
	Parvovirus infection		Infectious bronchitis
	Pasteurellosis		Infectious bursal disease (burnavirus)
	Swine erysipelas		Infectious laryngotracheitis
Horses	Equine abortion		Marek's disease
	Equine rhinopneumonitis		Newcastle disease
	Influenza	Dogs	Distemper
	Strangles		Infectious hepatitis
	Tetanus		Kennel cough complex
Cats	Calicivirus infection		Leptospirosis
	Leukaemia		Parvovirus
	Panleucopenia (parvovirus)		Rabies
	Rhinotracheitis (herpes virus)		

veterinary services due to economic, personnel or social problems, or occasionally due to the accidental importation of infected material.

The development of a very effective live attenuated (non-disease-causing) rinderpest vaccine by Walter Plowright in the 1950s made the control of rinderpest easier and it is predicted that the disease may be eliminated by 2010 and thereby become the first animal disease to be eliminated worldwide (Windsor, 2004). Unlike its predecessors, the Plowright vaccine (Anderson, 2004) could be used safely in all types of cattle of any age or health status. It could be produced very economically, and confers lifelong immunity.

The control of contagious bovine pleuropneumonia depended on isolation of individuals from herds, slaughter of individuals or herds, and quarantining farms, regions or countries. The slaughter of infected herds allowed the UK and USA to become clear of the disease in the early 1900s. Diagnostic tests, such as the complement fixation test developed in the 1930s, allowed the identification of infected animals not yet showing clinical signs of the disease and, combined with vaccines, they are now used in attempts to control the disease (Andrews and Windsor, 2004).

FMD is also controlled by isolation and quarantine, and vaccination programmes are used locally to control dissemination of the disease in countries in which FMD is endemic. In the 1940s, FMD was found worldwide. In 1996, endemic areas included Asia, Africa and parts of South America. Early vaccines used killed FMD virus to inoculate animals but there were sometimes problems with production of the vaccine which caused outbreaks in the 1970s, so scientists began making vaccines using only a single key protein from the virus. Whereas North America, Australia, New Zealand and Japan have been free of FMD for many years, most European countries have become disease-free more recently, and have discontinued vaccinating against the disease. In 2001, FMD in Britain resulted in the slaughter of many animals; there are arguments for and against the combination of slaughter and vaccination in controlling this disease (Kitching, 2004).

Bovine tuberculosis was a serious problem of dairy cows, and in the 1930s in the UK it was estimated that 40% of dairy cows were infected (Anonymous, 1965). Diagnostic tests using tuberculin to identify cattle infected with bovine tuberculosis were developed in the 1890s and were used in national testing schemes from the 1930s. Bovine tuberculosis control schemes have substantially reduced the incidence of this disease in cattle (Anonymous, 1965; Davidson, 2002).

Abortion due to brucellosis (*Brucella abortus*) was a major diseases problem of dairy cows until vaccines were first developed in the 1920s to prevent animals from aborting and until diagnostic tools were devised to identify infected animals (Anonymous, 1965). Brucellosis control programmes have now allowed many countries to eradicate the disease, such as New Zealand (Davidson, 2002). Likewise, clostridial diseases, for example blackleg, were important in cattle. They are now controlled largely by vaccines, the development of which began between 1910 and 1920. Nevertheless, it is instructive to note that even in developed nations these diseases will rapidly recur when veterinary intervention is thwarted. For instance, in Italy there were outbreaks of brucellosis in water buffalo, used in the production of mozzarella cheese, when local criminals reportedly intimidated and impeded the activities of local veterinarians (Fraser C, 2008).

Parasitic diseases
It is now also possible to control the major parasitic diseases of cattle, notably trypanosomiasis, anaplasmosis, babesiosis, East Coast fever, internal parasites, ticks

and tsetse flies (Robertson, 1976; Windsor, 2004), but problems may arise with maintaining control programmes and, more recently, with resistance to the anti-parasitic drugs in common use (Gopal *et al.*, 2001).

In Africa, tick and tsetse fly control programmes using a range of methodologies have allowed farmers and herdsmen to control trypanosomiasis and East Coast fever, respectively (Windsor, 2004). Tsetse fly control techniques include trapping using pheromones, use of insecticides and clearance of bush. Ixodicides to kill ticks have included arsenic, chlorinated hydrocarbons and organophosphates. Tick control is also important in controlling babesiosis and anaplasmosis. Effective anthelmintics have allowed the control of important internal parasites such as *Ostertagia* and liver fluke.

Additional diseases

Other bovine diseases are now controlled using antibiotics, for example mastitis, other treatments, for example hypocalcaemia and hypomagnesaemia, or a range of pharmaceuticals and management programmes (see Andrews, 2004). Many of these pharmaceuticals have been developed within the last half century.

3.3.3.2 Sheep

Two major veterinary developments have impacted greatly on lamb survival in the temperate farmlands of Australia, New Zealand, the UK and elsewhere. The first was the development, from the late 1940s, of effective cheap vaccines against clostridial diseases including pulpy kidney, tetanus, enterotoxaemia, dysentery, black disease, braxy and botulism, and the second was the development of effective anthelmintics which were first used in the 1960s (West *et al.*, 2002). Prior to the development of clostridial vaccines about one-third of growing lambs died.

The development of vaccines against other diseases has reduced their prevalence in sheep and improved welfare substantially. Vaccines are now available for a wide range of diseases of sheep (Table 3.3), all of which make disease control easier.

The development of effective drugs to treat internal and external parasites allowed the better utilization of extensive properties for sheep production. For instance, modern anthelmintics enabled the use of higher stocking densities by reducing the parasitic burden carried by closely stocked animals, and prevented sheep deaths from parasites such as *Haemonchus contortus* (barber's pole worm). The development of anthelmintic resistance in several species of internal parasite may have serious implications for the welfare of lambs, and until new anthelmintics or alternative methods of parasite control are developed high-density grazing of lambs will become more and more difficult. Efficient drugs, including chlorinated hydrocarbons, organophosphates and pyrethrins, to prevent and treat external parasites such as lice and flies, which cause myiasis or flystrike, were developed in the twentieth century. These chemicals have improved the quality of life of both sheep and shepherds. Sheep scab was eliminated in Australia and New Zealand in the early part of the twentieth century using dips of lime sulphur and arsenic, but continues to be a problem in the UK today.

3.3.3.3 Pigs

The intensification of pig-production systems warranted major improvements in the ability to control infectious diseases. Improved hygiene, the development of vaccines, the availability and use of antibiotics, and the practice of slaughtering infected herds helped combat major infectious diseases (Martin, 2000; McGlone and Pond, 2003; Kyriazakis and Whittemore, 2006; Table 3.3). Effective vaccines have reduced diseases such as Aujesky's disease, but improved management of sows and piglets is extremely important in disease control as is the maintenance of sound biosecurity systems (Kyriazakis and Whittemore, 2006). Internal parasites are easily controlled in pigs kept indoors, but treatment is required for pigs managed outdoors.

Despite major developments in veterinary science some pig diseases, such as hog cholera (classical swine fever), are still found in much of Asia, Latin America and parts of Africa and Europe. Australia, Britain, Canada, Ireland, New Zealand and Scandinavia are free of classical swine fever. Eradication is difficult and most programmes involve rapid diagnosis and culling, and emergency vaccination (Robertson, 1976).

3.3.3.4 Poultry

The development of vaccines against major poultry diseases in the 1940s and 1950s, for example Newcastle disease and infectious bronchitis, and the development of drugs to prevent coccidiosis, had a major impact on the health of poultry and allowed intensification of the poultry industry (Scanes et al., 2004). Vaccines for some diseases can now be given into the egg, provided in drinking water or sprayed on chicks, making delivery easy (see Appleby et al., 2004). In the UK in 1970, about 12% of hens would die during a laying cycle but this was reduced to 2–3% by 1990. Vaccination programmes combined with an 'all in all out' stocking policy, which allows for cleaning and disinfection between groups of birds, have contributed to this decline in mortality (Scanes et al., 2004). The intensification of poultry production has had a negative impact on poultry welfare in that laying hens are usually restricted in their ability to move around when caged and broilers are often managed in large flocks on deep litter. However, even with an anticipated introduction of better physical conditions for poultry in the future, their improved health will still depend on those developments in veterinary science mentioned above.

3.3.3.5 Horses

The misuse of working horses in developing countries and lack of effective veterinary care are important welfare issues (Wilson, 2002). However, the classic infectious disease of horses, strangles, can now be treated with antibiotics and controlled by vaccination and management (Newton and Chanter, 2003), and vaccines are also available for African horse sickness.

Veterinary understanding of the causes of lameness in horses has improved greatly through better diagnostic and imaging techniques which have allowed, during the last few decades, more accurate diagnosis and thereafter more directed treatment. Nevertheless, musculoskeletal injuries to sport and racing horses are important welfare issues causing pain and distress (Evans, 2002). Up to 40% of 2-year-old thoroughbred horses suffer from musculoskeletal injuries despite significant advances in the treatment of lameness (Mason and Bourke, 1973). A better understanding of the musculoskeletal development of young horses, an improved ability to identify the risk factors for such injuries (Perkins *et al.*, 2005) and greater knowledge of how training impacts on these will help reduce such problems in future.

Colic (abdominal pain) is a major problem in horses and although treatments for the range of causes of colic, including more effective analgesia and surgery, have improved greatly in the last two decades, the disease remains a significant problem for horses (see Robinson, 2003).

3.3.3.6 Companion animals
Vaccination and other control measures
Vaccine development against rabies, canine distemper, infectious canine hepatitis, leptospirosis, kennel cough and parvovirus disease have changed the health status of dogs worldwide (Table 3.3). In some developed countries, more than 95% of dogs are vaccinated, and distemper, hepatitis and leptospirosis, which were common, are now rare diseases (Stafford, 2006).

The eradication of rabies in some countries is a good example of the beneficial application of veterinary science. Rabies is a distressing fatal disease of warm-blooded animals, most especially dogs and humans. It was eliminated in Britain in 1922 following strict enforcement of dog control regulations; these allowed stray dogs to be picked up off the street and killed, forbade importation of dogs from abroad, and enforced the muzzling of all dogs on the street. The development of a vaccine against rabies allowed its use in a successful anti-rabies programme in Japan in 1921. An oral vaccine against rabies is now used to vaccinate wild animals against the disease.

The rapid development in the 1970s of a vaccine against parvovirus disease, shortly after it first appeared, bears testament to the advancement of veterinary science towards the latter half of the twentieth century. This new disease caused severe debility and/or high mortality in young puppies and was a major problem when first identified. General supportive treatment was effective if the disease was diagnosed early, but the rapid development of an effective vaccine contributed tremendously to reducing the incidence of the disease.

Improved methods of internal and external parasite control have greatly improved the welfare of cats and dogs, especially puppies. Modern flea-control methods such as the use of persistent topical solutions are much more effective than older techniques such as insecticide washes. Overall improvements in diet and health care, and promotion of indoor housing of cats in many countries mean that pet cats now routinely survive into their late teens (e.g. Lacheretz *et al.*, 2002), a previously rare occurrence.

Disposal of unwanted cats and dogs

A major welfare problem with cats and dogs is the production of unwanted kittens and puppies, as they either die from disease or starvation or are picked up and destroyed at animal shelters or animal control facilities. Some of these unplanned kittens and puppies are re-homed, but in most countries the majority die. It is estimated that each year about 20% of the dog population in the USA enter a shelter, and that half of these animals are killed (Stafford, 2006).

Veterinary contributions that have improved cat and dog population control include surgical de-sexing of young animals, hormonal contraception and immuno-contraception. The development of safe surgical de-sexing with good anaesthesia and analgesia, and de-sexing before the animals are re-homed, have markedly improved the humane management of unwanted kittens and puppies. Future developments in chemical and immunological sterilization techniques will contribute further, especially in developing countries where the facilities to surgically de-sex animals may not be available. The methods used to kill cats and dogs have also improved with the widespread use by veterinarians of the injectable anaesthetic pentobarbitone sodium.

Euthanasia of dogs

The development of a vaccine against rabies and effective treatment for ascarid worms of dogs may have influenced the relationship between people and dogs as people learned to be less afraid of them and more willing to enter into closer relationships with them. Veterinary science has nurtured this relationship by keeping dogs healthy and pain-free and increasing their longevity. However, advances in veterinary medicine and surgery now allow owners and veterinarians to keep alive animals that previously may have been euthanized. One of the major contemporary dilemmas facing veterinarians, therefore, is when to euthanize a companion animal and when to maintain it on palliative treatment. In one study of dogs, the majority that were euthanized by veterinarians were senile (60%) or suffered from terminal illness (27%), and only 2% were healthy (Edney, 1998). This suggests that euthanasia was being used appropriately, although the stage of senility or illness was not and probably could not easily be defined. Nevertheless, the close relationship between owner and companion animal and the greater surgical and medical options now available may result in animals being kept alive that would be better off dead.

The development of neuroactive drugs has also broadened the beneficial therapeutic contributions that veterinarians can make. Dogs with age-related cognitive dysfunction are now treated with drugs to reverse or slow their deterioration

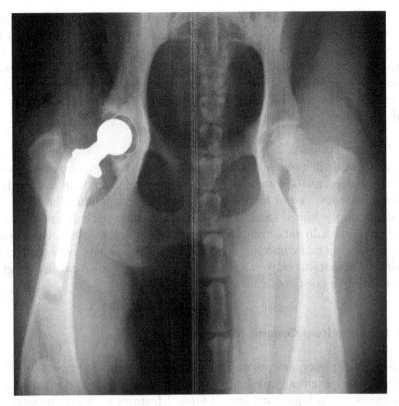

Figure 3.1 X-ray of a hip joint replacement in a dog (©2009, A.J. Worth, reproduced with permission).

and to prolong their lives. Dogs with serious anxiety problems are being treated pharmacologically, sometimes for their lifetime, and they may also be treated behaviourally to reduce the behaviours associated with anxiety. However, cautious evaluation of this practice would be advisable. The existence of anxious dogs suggests that problems may be present in the human–dog relationship, so that pharmacological treatments may mask inadequate management and environments.

Surgical developments and pain control

Developments in surgical procedures such as hip replacement (Figure 3.1) and kidney transplants have given veterinarians the ability to treat previously painful and incurable diseases and to lengthen and improve the quality of life. The pain caused by complicated orthopaedic surgery or chronic conditions such as some cancers can negatively affect the quality of life of the affected animal. The development of more effective analgesic protocols and of non-steroidal anti-inflammatory drugs and other analgesics has made pain alleviation much easier, and benefited the animals (Stafford, 2006). An increase in their use in cats and dogs has been particularly noticeable in the last few decades, both to treat surgical pain and pain caused by medical problems such as osteoarthritis. In the UK, it is estimated that about 1.3 million dogs of a total population of about 6 million suffer from osteoarthritis, and that about half of them are now treated. Pain relief is a substantial issue for the welfare of all species (Mellor *et al.*, 2008b) and the increased use of analgesics by veterinarians makes a significant difference to the lives of many animals, including cats and dogs.

3.3.3.7 Other animals

The developments in veterinary science in zoo animals, wildlife, other domestic animals (buffaloes, goats, camels, alpacas, llamas) and aviary and wild birds have been significant but are not listed. A major field of development has been in the areas of laboratory animal science. Much biomedical research depends on laboratory animals, especially rats, mice, guinea pigs, rabbits and hamsters. Developments in the management and control of disease in these species have been significant. In addition, the assessment of pain and its alleviation in these species has progressed significantly in the last two decades.

3.4 Learning from Organic Management

Here, aspects of the organic management of livestock are commented upon as a counterpoint to current approaches that include conventional veterinary support. The purposes are to highlight some additional features of the contributions veterinary care makes to livestock health and welfare, not dealt with above, or dealt with in other ways, and to draw attention to the possibility that rigorous scientific examination of the claimed benefits of organic management may reveal ways that veterinary therapies could be beneficially modified.

3.4.1 Before the advent of modern veterinary science all animal management was effectively organic

The major relevant difference between present day conventional and organic management of livestock is that organic precepts usually exclude the use of such things as vaccines, pharmaceuticals, insecticides and commercially manufactured fertilizers (Anonymous, 2001a). It is worth recalling, however, that use of such agents was introduced originally because of perceived inadequacies with the prior 'organic' approaches, and that, in general, their use has demonstrably improved animal productivity, health and welfare (see above). As is usual with any system, some disadvantages also emerged (see Chapter 1) and these are now advanced to justify the modern organic movement. These include contamination of food and the environment with harmful chemicals, and related concerns about human health and environmental sustainability. Also, benefits to animal welfare of adopting organic precepts are often mentioned, but usually as a secondary consideration.

3.4.2 Modern veterinary support was designed to minimize negative consequences of individual variability in animals farmed in large groups

Increasingly over the last 50 years veterinary and related scientific inputs into farm animal management have been developed to facilitate dealing with large numbers of animals in groups where opportunities to give attention to individuals are limited. Thus, preventative measures such as vaccination against tetanus or tail-docking lambs for flystrike reduction are applied to all animals, even when the proportion of those that might be adversely affected when not so protected would be fairly small. Although this means that many animals may be treated that do not require it, the strategy avoids the close surveillance that is needed to provide treatment to individuals only when they require it.

Individual variation in the biological responses of animals of the same species is normal so that some animals are more or less susceptible to particular welfare challenges than others, and their susceptibility may change from season to season or year to year. In a given on-farm situation, therefore, some animals in each herd or group may exhibit a degree of compromise in one or more of the five domains of welfare, and other animals may not. The proportion of animals exhibiting compromise is more likely to be greater when the on-farm conditions are poor and veterinary support of the type described above is not provided, than when such support is provided. Thus, veterinary support can in some cases compensate for otherwise suboptimal farm conditions. Regardless of this, more individual attention needs to be given to animals managed according to organic precepts if related deleterious effects on health and welfare are to be minimized (see below).

3.4.3 Aspects of disease control programmes might be omitted without problems, but some veterinary treatments will continue to be necessary

The complex aetiologies of many diseases allow for a variety of preventive programmes to be developed and may allow for specific aspects of any one complex control programme to be ignored or replaced without serious implications for the overall impact of the disease. To ascertain whether or not this is the case, however, each disease and the limitations imposed on treatment by the prohibitions of organic farming need to be evaluated separately. For instance, some alternative programmes may be effective in controlling conditions in dairy cows such as mastitis, clinical parasitism and lameness. If the incidence of these diseases can be maintained on organic farms at levels equal to or lower than on conventional farms then the welfare of the cows will not be adversely affected.

Nevertheless, in the absence of striking progress in genetic trait selection for disease resistance, it is clear that some major debilitating, distressing and fatal infectious diseases in farmed livestock will not be able to be controlled without vaccination (Table 3.3). It is also clear that for some diseases success without vaccine use on individual farms may result from low exposure to the infectious agents because neighbouring farmers will still vaccinate their stock. Likewise, severe internal or external parasitic infestations, for example haemonchosis and flystrike, will require veterinary treatment with effective anti-parasitic remedies if protracted debility, pain or death are to be avoided. Finally, injuries or other conditions requiring remedial surgery, or other health conditions and husbandry practices that cause significant and treatable pain, can only be managed appropriately with the use of anaesthetics and/or analgesics. Any purposeful avoidance of such proven remedies that results in serious health and welfare compromise would be a matter of significant concern.

3.4.4 Greater knowledge, skill and attention to individual animals is required when veterinary support is withdrawn

Managing animals without modern veterinary support demands meticulous attention to the details of the usually multi-faceted methods that are then required to maintain healthy and productive animals. This also means that the staff require greater knowledge and skill to recognize problems before they become serious. Numerous features of the management of health and welfare conditions are often the same on conventional and organic farms, although greater care is required on organic farms which do not have the safety margins afforded by 'chemical-based' veterinary inputs. For instance, management programmes to reduce the incidence of mastitis on dairy farms list about 30 recommendations and only two of these, dry cow therapy and treatment of clinical cases using antibiotics, are not permitted by organic dairy farm codes (Brightling *et al.*, 1998; Anonymous, 1999). A severe culling programme of affected cows during lactation, careful and frequent milking-machine maintenance, frequent rubber replacement, good milking practice, teat-spraying or -dipping, environmental cleanliness, the use of teat sealants at drying-off, lower stocking density and attempts to increase immunocompetence before calving by increasing selenium, zinc and vitamin E levels may all play a part in reducing the incidence of mastitis. In order to manage mastitis, most organic farmers use the majority of these conventional management practices combined with alternative therapy.

3.4.5 Application of organic precepts may reveal areas where some 'chemical-based' veterinary remedies can be avoided without compromising animal health and welfare

With any management system it is possible to become locked into deploying long-standing routines because they have not been refreshed by critical re-examination after their initial introduction. Applying a dictum of complete or substantial withdrawal of 'chemical-based' veterinary remedies has the potential, therefore, to reveal not only those practices that are essential (see above) but also those that are over-used or can be avoided because the condition being treated can be legitimately and efficiently managed in other ways. So the organic challenge to conventional livestock management may well reveal improvements that conventional farmers would wish to apply.

Unfortunately, as yet there is a dearth of rigorous research into the development of effective disease management and control on organic farms and into how organic systems, when successful, result in reasonably low levels of, for instance, infectious disease and parasitism. Further research into comparing animal health, welfare and productivity on paired organic and conventional farms would provide greater understanding of what happens on the former. For instance, there are different types of organic farm, and comparison should be made between them especially during the transition period from conventional to organic approaches when serious health and welfare problems can occur (Weller and Bowling, 2000; Mackay, 2001). Also, it may be important for organic farmers to develop management programmes and production targets quite different from conventional farms and to define when conventional veterinary remedies must be used to maintain animal welfare. This clearly can be effective in some circumstances, as the available data suggest, for instance, that dairy cattle on organic farms are often no worse off than dairy cattle on conventional farms (McDonald et al., 1994; Weller and Cooper, 1996; Hamilton et al., 2002). Finally, it is worth noting that the ranges of animal welfare standards on conventional and organic farms may be similar, so that restricted use of veterinary remedies does not automatically mean that health and welfare will be compromised unacceptably, but, as already noted, avoiding major problems may often require higher levels of knowledge and skill, and a much stronger commitment to managing the stock as individuals.

There is very little evidence from science-based research to show that alternative therapies are effective in the treatment or control of livestock diseases. Thus, although textbooks on the use of homeopathy (MacLeod, 1964; Verkade, 1997), acupuncture (Rogers and Janssens, 1991) and herbalism (de Bairacli Levy, 1953) in livestock are available, there are few peer-reviewed publications in the veterinary literature demonstrating the efficacy of these alternative or complementary approaches. Indeed, concerns have been raised in human medicine about the potential toxic side effects of some herbal treatments (Abbott et al., 1996; Carter, 1996). It is important to remember that conventional farmers would welcome the development of therapies and prophylactic systems which do not involve antibiotics, for instance, because antibiotic use results in milk having to be discarded and withholding times that delay presentation for slaughter. The use of alternative therapies becomes a welfare issue when the diseases or injuries being treated are causing distress or pain and the alternative therapy does not work as effectively and as quickly as scientifically proven treatments.

3.5 The Future

3.5.1 Past achievements show that further marked improvements in animal health and welfare are likely

The veterinary developments of the twentieth century were profound and in the main have improved the welfare of animals significantly. It is likely that ongoing developments in the twenty-first century will continue at the rate seen in the previous 100 years, and we can expect major further reductions of disease and pain in all domestic animals. It is possible that animals will routinely be subjected to mass diagnostic tests which will allow earlier detection of problems and earlier treatment using a much wider suite of therapies than are available today. These will most likely include remote monitoring of animals for disease notification and gene therapy (Beall *et al.*, 2000). However, the use of veterinary developments that improve production must be tempered with the need to maintain and improve the welfare of livestock and poultry.

One major problem that requires attention is the alleviation of pain in livestock subjected to standard husbandry practices such as castration, tail-docking and disbudding or dehorning (Mellor *et al.*, 2008b). Improvements may be achieved by reducing the need for such practices, but pain alleviation will also receive attention. Some older common problems are still major causes of poor welfare in livestock and these include footrot in sheep, lameness as well as mastitis and metabolic problems in dairy cattle, and colic in horses. But there are also modern problems, such as obesity in cats and dogs, which result from improved nutrition, and hereditary problems which may result from keeping animals alive which are physically compromised to unacceptable levels or that are incapable of reproducing naturally. The development of the Belgian Blue cattle breed, which relies on Caesarean section for calving, is a case where veterinary skills have allowed the selection of abnormal physical states. A similar situation with many breeds of dogs is equally questionable, where, for instance, Caesarean sections may be required in 62% of Boston terriers and 43% of French bulldogs (Linde-Forsberg, 2001). In such cases, a 'can-do' attitude with regard to technical capability appears to have swamped common sense and our ethical obligation to minimize the harm we do to animals as we apply our ever-increasing knowledge and skills to manipulating them to serve our human purposes (Fisher and Mellor, 2008).

Genetics, Biotechnology and Animal Breeding

Mixed Blessings

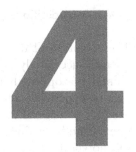

4.1 Introduction

The evolution of different animal species, it is believed, has equipped them to operate successfully in their particular ecological niche. Thus, the ability of each animal to cope with its environment is influenced by genetics (its genotype), plus its experience and the environment. The genotype of domestic animals is a product of natural and artificial selection through domestication, breed development and ongoing selection for particular physical or behavioural attributes (phenotypes). Selection for particular phenotypic characteristics may be beneficial for a species, but it may also impact negatively on the physical capabilities, health and welfare of individual animals in their domesticated environment. It is anticipated that in the near future it will become easier to identify the genetic factors that may affect the physical and behavioural attributes of animals, and thereby to improve the selection of particular animals for breeding aimed at enhancing the health and welfare of domestic animals. The present chapter is directed at considering these matters.

4.2 A Brief History of Animal Breeding

4.2.1 Domestication and early breeding focused on physical features and temperament

The selection of animals to be used as breeding stock to produce offspring suited to particular human requirements is an ancient practice which began during the domestication of wild animals and birds and continued without any scientific understanding for thousands of years. This process, coupled with natural selection, resulted in animal types being produced which suited particular environments and human needs. Thus, many of the physical and behavioural characteristics of domesticated animals have resulted from this artificial selection based primarily on human preferences for particular phenotypic characteristics.

The pedigrees of particular lines of animals were documented in ancient times, but the major development of breeds has occurred during the last 500 years, and many breeds of farm and companion animals were produced in the eighteenth and nineteenth centuries. Coates' *Shorthorn Herd Book*, dated around 1800, was the first cattle breed book in Britain (Porter, 1991). Breed development occurred by placing selection emphasis on consistent identifiable physical characteristics and behavioural disposition; that is, a tractable temperament. Thus, size, shape, colour, hair or wool type, horn type and other obvious features were selected for, and only those animals with the desired characteristics were allowed into the breed book and could be used for breeding. By this means, many distinctive breeds of animals were produced without any understanding of how these characteristics were inherited.

4.2.2 The science of genetics enhanced breeding for particular characteristics

Our scientific understanding of genetics originated in the pioneering work of Gregor Mendel in the nineteenth century (Nicholas, 1996), whose work was carried out after many if not most of the common breeds of farm and companion animals had been developed. During the last century, major developments in genetic knowledge occurred and these accelerated as the genomes of different species were identified and our ability to identify quantitative trait loci (QTLs) related to specific characteristics became possible. Thus, although many of the livestock breeds produced in the nineteenth century are still important today, our greater understanding of genetics has allowed the production of new breeds, and lines within breeds, with particular characteristics suited to particular modern demands.

4.2.3 Science-based breeding has produced problems and may provide solutions

Paralleling the early emphasis on appearance was a desire to improve productivity, so that, for many years now, livestock and poultry selection indices have concentrated on increasing production and efficiency, a process which was aided by our burgeoning understanding of genetics (see McGlone and Pond, 2003). This selection direction allowed for some adaptation to the environmental changes, both physical and social, which occurred as production technologies developed. Nevertheless, ongoing selection for a limited number of production traits led to identifiable physical or behavioural problems (Grandin and Deesing, 1998a). Thus, the use of genetic knowledge to increase productivity often occurred without consideration of other important traits. However, more recent improvements in our understanding should now allow us to direct the power of genetic selection towards correcting such problems and also towards improving the health and welfare of production animals in the modern farming context.

Whereas modern livestock and poultry breeders have focused on production parameters and tended to reduce their prior emphasis on the shape and colour of their breeds, dog and cat breeders have taken the opposite approach (Stafford, 2006). They have stopped breeding for function and have exaggerated the physical standards of many breeds, often with deleterious consequences for their health and welfare. For instance, the breeding of dogs to meet such standards has produced many pedigree breeds that have a suite of hereditary problems and diseases (McGreevy and Nicholas, 1999). Fortunately, this situation can now be corrected. Developments in our understanding of how these problems are inherited, together with genetic screening of breeding animals for some of the important diseases, will allow the selection of healthy animals for breeding purposes. In addition, the development of gene-based therapies will allow for better treatment of some of these diseases (Beall *et al.*, 2000).

Table 4.1 Stages in a structured breeding programme (adapted from McGlone and Pond, 2003).

Stage	Action
1	Identify and define the objective of the programme
2	Choose selection criteria
3	Develop a pedigree scheme
4	Develop a performance-recording scheme
5	Evaluate breeding values: use the best linear unbiased predictor
6	Use marker-assisted selection
7	Identify animals for breeding

4.3 Modern Livestock Breeds and Breeding

Human demand for livestock-based products changes over time and livestock may be farmed in environments unlike those in which their breeds were developed. Also, there is persistent pressure to keep production costs down. Geneticists respond by using a basic breeding programme (Table 4.1) to produce new strains or breeds that better meet these requirements. They may quantify the heritability of different characteristics of animals and this determines how easily specific characteristics can be bred for or against. Within-breed selection may be too slow to allow for the desired changes, and the production of new breeds may be more efficient (Nicholas, 1996).

The development of 'new' animal types in these ways can improve welfare if the animals are better suited to the production environment, or it can reduce welfare if there is a mismatch between their specific and sometimes different requirements for health and welfare and what can be provided from the environment. It is convenient to consider such animal welfare outcomes by making reference to the nutritional, environmental, health and behavioural needs of animals, although it should be noted that there is often some degree of overlap. As noted in Chapter 1, not meeting the animals' needs in these four domains may be registered in the fifth, mental, domain in terms of unpleasant experiences the animal may have, and meeting their needs will result in neutral or good experiences. Examples of some negative and positive animal welfare consequences of breeding for specific traits are provided below.

4.3.1 Nutrition: breeding-induced high productivity can outstrip nutrient supply

Nutrients in food are required for maintenance of the body's structure and background functions. They are also required for additional metabolically demanding activities such as exercise, heat production when in cold environments, pregnancy, growth, and for milk, fibre (wool or hair) and egg production. When the genotype of a strain or breed of animal exaggerates functions such as growth or milk production, nutrient demand can be precariously balanced with nutrient supply to the detriment of the animal's welfare in the short or long term, or both.

4.3.1.1 Consequences of high growth rate of broiler (meat) chickens

The growth rate and feed-use efficiency of broilers has doubled since the 1940s so that now a chicken can grow from a 45-g 1-day-old bird to 2200 g or more 42 days later (Appleby *et al.*, 2004). The selection for rapid growth of broilers puts them at a risk of lameness, and a large proportion of juvenile birds and males retained for breeding become lame. In some studies, up to 30% of broilers have some abnormal gait. The poultry industry is now selecting for reduced lameness (Appleby *et al.*, 2004) but *lameness* remains a major problem in broiler chicks. Lameness can be kept at much lower levels than this by strict biosecurity (to avoid infections), and dietary and environmental strategies. Juvenile broiler chickens are allowed to eat *ad libitum*, thus satisfying appetite, until taken for slaughter at 35–45 days of age, but broilers used for breeding are fed 60–80% *less* than they would eat during growth, and 50% *less* during egg laying (see Grandin and Deesing, 1998b). Thus they would be chronically hungry.

4.3.1.2 Thinness and metabolic burnout in high-producing dairy cows

Breeding of dairy cows directed at increasingly high milk production has transformed the relationship of the udder to the rest of the body. Previously, the udder was an appendage to the body such that its metabolic demands were secondary and milk production would usually decrease in times of scarce feed supply. Now, in some breeds the udder takes precedence when nutrients are being partitioned between milk production and other body functions, so that milk production drains nutrients from the body when feed supply is inadequate. Such animals are more vulnerable to day-to-day variations in nutrient availability and easily become very thin, and presumably hungry, during feed shortages. There may be long-term detrimental effects which are reflected in the need to cull such animals due to reproductive problems after only two or three lactations, compared with about eight lactations in lower-producing breeds. The emphasis on breeding for milk yield has produced other problems, such as an increased tendency towards lameness in Holstein cattle.

4.3.2 Environment: breeding for 'environmental fit' can improve welfare

The traditional European breeds of cattle and sheep were developed in temperate latitudes with moderate ambient temperatures and generally sufficient rainfall for adequate grass production. These breeds, particularly some from Britain, were taken by colonists to Africa, the Americas and Oceania, where conditions were often quite different. The welfare, health and productivity of these breeds were often compromised as they were exposed to air temperatures, relative humidity, forages and parasites unlike those of their original environment. New breeds were therefore produced in Australia and the USA by crossing European with tropical breeds. The characteristics required included heat tolerance, suitable coat colour and type, large and more numerous sweat glands, and parasite tolerance. Crosses of *Bos taurus* and *Bos indicus* cattle, for instance, have the production values of the former and the heat tolerance and tick resistance of the latter (Nicholas, 1996), so that breeds such as the Droughtmaster and Australian Milking Zebu (Williamson and Payne, 1978), in being better suited to the climate, could also meet production requirements. This experience showed that such attributes could be identified and selected for to produce breeds more suited to tropical conditions.

The understanding of how to identify suitable selection criteria, quantify the hereditability of desirable characteristics and measure breeding values is now regarded as basic genetics and has been deployed with some success. For instance, during the last 50 years this knowledge helped the introduction of sheep and cattle to land not previously used for such production. In New Zealand, the Perendale sheep breed, developed from Romney and Cheviot stock, was better suited to large sheep farms on rough hill country because it foraged widely and was more mobile than its antecedents (Whateley *et al.*, 1974). In the USA, beef breeds such as the Charbray and Santa Gerturdis, both crosses of European (Charolais and Shorthorn, respectively) and Brahman stock, were bred to suit particular physical environments (Porter, 1991).

Crossbreeding continues to be a useful tool for contemporary livestock production. Thus, in New Zealand Friesian and Jersey dairy breeds are crossbred to produce an animal which is thought to be hardier and more suited to the type of dairy farming currently practised there (Holmes *et al.*, 2002). Likewise in the UK, the sheep industry is based around a number of breeds which are crossbred to produce varieties suited to particular environments and needs.

4.3.3 Health: breeding can eliminate genetic disorders and increase disease resistance

4.3.3.1 Elimination of genetic disorders

Good health is fundamental to good welfare, and veterinary developments over the last century have improved animal health markedly (Mellor and Bayvel, 2008; Chapter 3). Although much of this improvement has occurred with the development of vaccines and effective pharmaceuticals to prevent or treat disease, other diseases are inherited (Table 4.2). The identification of heritable diseases in livestock and companion animals, and their means of inheritance, have enabled the development of programmes which allow for the elimination of specific diseases from animal populations. The key to these programmes is the deployment of objective criteria which can be used easily to identify clinically normal but genetically affected animals. Two examples of success stories in livestock are described below.

Table 4.2 The four modes of inheritance of diseases (adapted from Oberbauer and Sampson, 2001).

Mode of inheritance	Features
Autosomal dominant	The gene is found as a heterozygous and not a homozygous state Males and females are equally affected One parent of affected animals has the disease If one parent is heterozygous then about 50% of offspring are affected
Autosomal recessive	Affected animals are homozygous for the gene If healthy, both parents of affected offspring are heterozygous carriers Males and females are equally affected
Polygenic	Erratic appearance of disease Both males and females are affected but the proportion affected may vary There are no predictable ratios in pedigrees because the number of genes involved unknown
Sex-linked recessive	The characteristic pattern of transmission is that female offspring are normal and male offspring are affected Affected males have no affected sons and carrier daughters

Alpha-mannosidosis

This disease causes ataxia in calves at birth, and is due to a deficiency of lysosomal α-mannosidase. Affected animals have little of this enzyme, but heterozygotes have one normal and one mutant gene and about half the normal enzyme activity (Jolly, 2002). An enzyme test which identified heterozygotes that were otherwise normal was the basis of a programme in New Zealand to eliminate the disease from the pedigree Aberdeen Angus herd.

Spider lamb syndrome

Hereditary chondrodysplasia (spider lamb syndrome) is a disease of Suffolk and Hampshire sheep caused by an autosomal recessive gene, resulting in long, bent limbs. A DNA test which determines whether sheep have the hereditary chondrodysplasia gene is available. If positive, animals are not used for breeding the disease will disappear (West *et al.*, 2002).

4.3.3.2 Breeding for disease resistance or tolerance

Consumer concern about the use of antibiotics, hormones and other drugs in food animals has put pressure on livestock producers to employ alternative techniques to prevent disease in animals. However, the elimination or reduction in drug use, without the development of alternative disease prevention or treatment protocols, may cause welfare problems (Chapter 3). There is thus growing interest in breeding for resistance or tolerance to important infectious diseases, such as avian influenza (Doran and Lambeth, 2007), or to diseases caused by internal or external parasites.

Nevertheless, there are many difficulties in producing strains of livestock that are resistant or tolerant to different viruses, bacteria or parasites (Tellam, 2007). The genetic variation underlying disease resistance may be complex, probably combining gene–gene and gene–environment interactions (Tellam, 2007). Other problems in breeding for disease resistance include identification of objective criteria and environmental effects. However, there have been some successes.

Bacterial infection

Although disease resistance may involve more than one gene (polygenic) it may be inherited in a simple fashion, as illustrated by resistance to neonatal diarrhoea caused by *Escherichia coli* K88 in piglets. The receptor on the wall of the piglet's intestine, which binds with the K88 antigen, is the result of a dominant gene. Piglets that are homogenous or heterogenous for this gene have the receptor, so that K88 can bind to the intestine, and diarrhoea may develop. Piglets with the recessive gene do not have the receptor and are therefore not susceptible to diarrhoea caused by these bacteria (see Nicholas, 1996).

Parasitic infections

In pastoral livestock systems, anti-parasitic drugs have been essential in allowing more intensive grazing by livestock. Resistance to anthelmintics and insecticides is a growing problem and one of the proposed alternatives is to breed animals that are resistant to or tolerant of the parasites these drugs target. In addition, the cost and availability of drugs to livestock producers in many African countries, where parasitic diseases of cattle are a major problem, makes the development of resistant strains important for both animal and human welfare. Research into the development of resistant or tolerant strains of livestock is ongoing, but to date there have been few successes.

Flystrike, or myiasis, occurs when blowfly larvae consume areas of skin and underlying tissues of living animals. One programme in New Zealand to produce sheep resistant to myiasis has concentrated on breeding sheep with short tails and virtually no wool in the perineal area (Scobie *et al.*, 1999). As most cases of flystrike occur in response to flies laying their eggs in accumulations of urine-soaked faecal pads attached to perineal wool, sheep with little or no wool in that area are likely to be less attractive to the flies that cause myiasis. Public disquiet regarding the painful practice of mulesing Merino sheep in Australia, a practice designed to reduce flystrike by surgically reducing perineal wool, has given impetus to the breeding of Merinos with appropriately modified perineal skin and wool characteristics.

Resistance to facial eczema

The development of strains of sheep resistant to facial eczema is a major issue in New Zealand. Facial eczema is a disease of ruminants which follows ingestion of spores of a pasture fungus (*Pithomyces chartarum*). The spores release a toxin, sporidesmin, resulting in liver damage. The heritability for susceptibility to facial eczema in sheep is 0.42, which is high and indicates that breeding for low susceptibility is possible (Smith and Towers, 2002). The criterion for resistance used is the γ-glutamyltransferase (GGT) response of rams given a challenge dose of sporidesmin. Resistant rams show little or no response in plasma GGT, and if used for breeding they increase the proportion of resistant animals in a flock. A genetic marker for resistance is sought.

Genetic markers and the future
Development of strains of resistant animals would be facilitated by the identification of genetic markers for resistance. The results to date with diseases such as bovine mastitis are encouraging. Somatic cell counts are a good criterion for mastitis and are heritable. Artificial breeding is usual in well-developed dairy industries, and if bulls with a trait to resist mastitis are identified this characteristic would be easily spread.

4.3.4 Behaviour: breeding for desired behavioural attributes and temperament is possible
Deliberate selection for particular behavioural characteristics has been undertaken successfully for many years. Characteristics successfully selected for include strong maternal behaviour in some sheep breeds (Fraser and Broom, 1990), ease of milk letdown in dairy cows (Goddard and Wiggans, 1999) and the great variety of behavioural attributes in different dog breeds (Stafford, 2006). These observations indicate, in addition, that the behaviour of any one species has potential to be modified substantially in many different ways by selection for particular attributes. Indeed, some behaviours have been shown quantitatively to be highly hereditable. In dairy cows, for instance, where ease of milk letdown, speed of milking, temperament and the 'likeability' of the animals are preferred attributes, heritability for milking speed has been estimated to be 0.21–0.25, temperament about 0.16 and 'likeability' about 0.20 (Goddard and Wiggans, 1999). Some heritability estimates for temperament are even higher, being between 0.4 and 0.5 in dairy and beef cattle, respectively (see Grandin and Deesing, 1998b). Thus, it should be relatively easy to select for animals that have a quiet, docile and confident temperament with low levels of aggression and fear, thereby further enhancing their welfare in the farm environment.

Behaviour illustrates how animals cope with their environment. This includes close contact with stock handlers and even the different attitudes and behaviour these people have towards the animals (see Hemsworth and Coleman, 1998; Chapters 7 and 9). This is perhaps especially the case with intensively managed livestock. Thus, it may be anticipated that some selective breeding for the ability to cope with intensive-housing systems, or with forced inactivity, probably occurs inevitably when selecting for increased production and improved feed conversion in such systems. However, deliberate selection for the ability to cope with restrictive or barren environments, such as in layer-hen cages or sow stalls, has not been undertaken. If such breeding were to be pursued it would be of paramount importance to identify behaviours that would provide convincing evidence of improved welfare status, and not simply the appearance of improvement (Beausoleil *et al.*, 2008). Although this is feasible, the ethical question of whether or not selection for these purposes should be undertaken at all needs to be addressed.

Some animals may be predisposed to express abnormal behaviours, and this may be inherited. If so, it would be possible to breed away from them, but this could reduce the animal's behavioural repertoire, and this may limit their ability to cope with inadequate environments. Nevertheless, if genetic components of cannibalism, feather-pecking and aggression in poultry were to be bred out, better welfare would result from elimination of the associated pain and distress. Feather-pecking is probably polygenic, and separate QTLs for it at 6 and 30 weeks of age have been identified, which suggests that selection against it may be possible using marker-assisted selection. If selection against feather-pecking were to be successful it would also make beak-trimming unnecessary, thereby eliminating any pain and distress associated with that procedure. On the other hand, although pre-laying pacing and agitation in layer hens may reflect frustration of some sort, it is not clear that selecting against this behaviour would improve their welfare because of uncertainties about appropriate behavioural indices of frustration or its absence (Appleby *et al.*, 2004).

The prospect of breeding for specific behavioural responses to improve animal welfare allows the imagination to run. For example, could sheep be produced that are afraid of dogs and thus allow mustering, but at ease with humans and thus allow close contact, say during lambing? Although this might be possible, it should be noted that not all behaviours, normal or abnormal, are likely to be amenable to genetic modification. For instance, rumination is such a fundamental behaviour that it may not be possible to breed ruminants that are content to ruminate less when fed indoors, but revert to normal behaviour when returned to pasture. Thus, sheep held indoors and fed inadequate roughage are likely to continue plucking wool from other sheep in order to evoke rumination.

Notwithstanding the many breeding successes to date, advancing the science of behavioural genetics, which is in its infancy, is at present hindered by several problems. These include the following: (1) it is difficult to separate the impact of post-conception experience and environment from the effects of genotype; (2) behaviour is technically difficult to measure and measured parameters often do not conform to a normal distribution, thereby complicating statistical evaluations; (3) interpreting the biological significance of different behaviours is sometimes problematical; (4) livestock have long intergenerational intervals, few offspring and are late reaching social maturity; (5) behaviours may be exhibited infrequently and may be influenced by learning and social circumstances and (6) many behaviours are polygenic, and this increases the difficulty of selecting for and against them. In the long term, however, these current impediments do not seem to be insurmountable.

4.4 Companion Animals

4.4.1 Inbreeding for exaggerated physical attributes that has harmed some dog and cat breeds must be corrected

Dog breeders have tended to exaggerate the physical characteristics of their breeds and have developed breed standards which emphasize those attributes. The prior functional competence and health of earlier representatives of individual dog breeds, for example, have often been harmed in this selection process. Thus, breeds that were once athletic and aggressive have become physically compromised and non-aggressive. The change in the English Bulldog over the last two centuries graphically illustrates this (Figure 4.1). These extreme characteristics and attendant health and

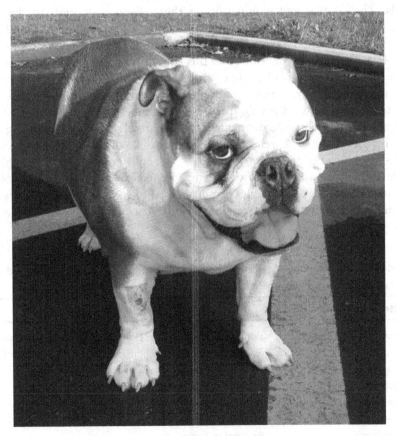

Figure 4.1 English Bulldog (©2009, A.J. Worth, reproduced with permission).

welfare problems could be easily reversed by breed societies changing their breed standards, so that breeders would be motivated to select breeding animals with less extreme characteristics. Of course, it has already been noted that such breeding has not been limited to companion animals, as physical features have also been exaggerated in some livestock and poultry breeds to their detriment, for example Belgian Blue cattle, broiler chickens and turkeys.

Many breeds of pedigree dogs have long lists of heritable diseases (Padgett, 1998), and overall there are more than 1050 inherited disorders in dogs, about half of which are inherited by a simple monogenic means (Giger *et al.*, 2006). Much of the last two centuries of dog breeding has involved genetic isolation and inbreeding, and only a few animals were used in the development of many breeds. Within a breed, the success in the show ring of individual male champions and their subsequent wide use as breeding animals reduced the gene pool even further. This breeding strategy greatly increased the incidence of heritable diseases and although this was not deliberate it was an inevitable outcome of persistent line breeding and has major welfare implications for the affected animals. The control and elimination of these diseases depends on knowing how each disease is inherited and how to identify affected animals. Giger *et al.* (2006) list the hereditary disorders characterized at the molecular genetic level (Table 4.3). Control also depends, and this is important, on strong support from concerned breed clubs, and if that is not forthcoming, legislation should be considered. Fortunately, genetic counselling (Fowler *et al.*, 2000) by geneticists and veterinarians now offers the prospect that inherited diseases can be controlled and perhaps eliminated. Such counselling involves defining breeding goals for the breeder, identifying relevant inherited diseases of the breed, gathering the knowledge of how the diseases are inherited, and collecting genotypic and phenotypic data about the animal's relatives. The outcomes of various mating strategies are then calculated, and strategies are developed to maximize healthy offspring while maintaining the good aspects of the different bloodlines (Oberbauer and Sampson, 2001).

Table 4.3 Some hereditary diseases of dog breeds which have been characterized at the genetic level (adapted from Giger *et al.*, 2006).

Hereditary disease	Breeds affected
von Willebrand disease type I	Bernese Mountain dogs, Doberman Pinscher, Kerry Blue Terrier, Manchester Terrier, Papillon, Pembroke Welsh Corgi, Poodles, West Highland Terrier
von Willebrand disease type II	German Shorthaired and Wirehaired Pointers
von Willebrand disease type III	Scottish Terrier
Mucopolysaccharidosis type IIIA	Wirehaired Dachshund, New Zealand Huntaway
Copper toxicosis	Bedlington Terrier

4.5 Breeding Technologies

4.5.1 Artificial insemination (AI) has been, and is, a very mixed blessing

The development of AI for a number of mammalian and avian species was a major breakthrough in animal agriculture as it allowed individual male animals with particularly valuable features to be used as sires over many more females than would have been possible naturally. This technology has had positive and negative consequences with regard to the welfare of the species involved.

In general, artificial breeding programmes concentrated on economically important features such as milk production, growth or meat production. In some cases this emphasis, combined with widespread use of particular animals, promulgated phenotypes which had particular deficiencies, resulting in poorer welfare than in existing livestock. For instance, there was a greater susceptibility of high-producing dairy cows to lameness and mastitis. In other cases, ready uptake of AI also led to improved animal welfare. Thus, it gave dairy and beef farmers on small holdings, for example, immediate access to better-quality bulls, which probably improved the physical characteristics and health of their livestock, and allowed them to stop keeping bulls which were often of dubious quality and managed inappropriately.

The mixed blessing of AI may be illustrated in another way. The widespread use of semen from any individual animal may allow the rapid spread within a species of unwanted or adverse characteristics. Concentrating on milk yield, for example, may allow the use of bulls with conformational characteristics which make cows more susceptible to lameness. However, the reverse is also true. Desirable inherited characteristics, such as resistance to mastitis or conformation which prevents lameness, could be spread throughout a national herd of cattle quickly and easily. The greater understanding of this now will help to ensure that future artificial breeding will be used to disseminate physical and behavioural characteristics that are known to improve welfare.

AI has also had both positive and negative effects because it has eliminated the need for copulation. Thus, on the negative side it has allowed the breeding of turkeys of such a large size that AI is now essential if they are to breed, and its use in dogs allows the production of offspring with physical or behavioural characteristics that would otherwise preclude natural mating. On the positive side, the use of AI in some horse breeds eliminates the need to keep stallions isolated and to expect them to mate with large numbers of mares unknown to them. The isolation of stallions and exposure to unknown mares is unnatural, and many mares have to be restrained to prevent them kicking the stallion.

An important welfare problem with pedigree dogs is the very limited number of animals of breeds that are not particularly popular in any country. Access to unrelated breeding animals is difficult and the importation of new animals may be expensive and limited for biosecurity reasons; that is, to prevent cross-border spread of animal diseases. The collection, storage and international transportation of canine semen allows for new blood lines to be imported and for outbreeding to occur much more effectively than via importation of animals. Careful scrutiny of the dog from which semen is collected is important, as the presence of inherited diseases and defects in that dog could detrimentally affect the national population of that breed. However, the alternative strategy of using semen from many dogs from different blood lines of the same breed would allow breeders to select in favour of physical and behavioural health, and away from heritable diseases.

4.5.2 Embryo transfer and cloning can be beneficial if we learn lessons from AI

The development of embryo transfer had similar effects to AI, but in contrast to AI, which promulgates male characteristics, embryo transfer allowed the genes of individual female animals to be multiplied. Broadly, the procedure is that donor eggs are obtained by superovulation. After fertilization, they are then transplanted into recipient animals, 'surrogate mothers', which give birth at the end of pregnancy and rear the offspring as their own. Embryo transfer has been used to increase the number of animals of particular breeds and for international movement of particular breeds or strains of animals. As with AI, incautious use of embryo transfer could easily multiply phenotypes with animal welfare problems, such as the transfer of European breeds of cattle or sheep to a climate or environment to which they are unsuited. However, it is usually used to increase the opportunities for farmers to improve the quality of their livestock, including enhancing animal welfare status.

Artificial breeding programmes that allow selection of the sex of offspring in dairy cattle will become economically worthwhile in the future. Selection of female and male offspring would allow the destruction of unwanted Jersey bull calves to be reduced and could permit the production of beef-type crossbred calves which are male or female as required. Such selection may also reduce the need for rearing Friesian bull calves, with their attendant behavioural and intraspecific aggression problems.

The recent development of cloning of sheep, cattle, horses, dogs and cats allows the extensive multiplication of very similar individual animals. It has important possibilities for biomedical research but is not likely to become a significant animal agricultural procedure in the near future (Wells and Laible, 2007). Companion animals and horses are being cloned for owners who want a new animal reasonably similar to a previous pet or athlete. There are some problems with cloning and 30% of the calves conceived by nuclear transfer had abnormalities such as excessive fetal growth, prolonged gestation and joint problems (see Smidt and Niemann, 1999). Indeed, only 64% of cloned calves survived to weaning (Wells et al., 2004). Also, the annual mortality rate in adult cloned cattle (8%) was much higher than that of normal animals (Wells et al., 2004). However, many cloned animals are physiologically normal and improvements in techniques will probably reduce issues surrounding mortality.

Transgenesis – the insertion of additional genes into the genome – in livestock will probably focus on animal production, disease resistance, meat and milk quality and specific products, for example medicines, to be produced in milk, and environmental suitability (Wells and Laible, 2007). The development of methodologies to utilize our rapidly developing knowledge in this area will impact on the welfare of the species involved. The effect of these developments on the welfare of production animals remains unclear and will continue to be so until they are used more widely. There are obvious positive and negative outcomes of transgenesis but the overall results remain uncertain.

4.6 The Future

Molecular genetics is a rapidly developing science. It has the potential to revolutionize the breeding of animals to better suit them to a wide range of environments and uses by providing them with, for instance, greater resistance to major parasitic and infectious diseases, and with temperaments that include generally high thresholds for aggression and anxiety, all of which would improve animal welfare. Additional areas likely to receive attention include selection for improved production, for example improved feed efficiency, and more desirable or marketable products, for example carcass quality, while retaining or developing characteristics that promote animal welfare. Such breeding is likely to be based increasingly on genomic profiles rather than progeny testing as our knowledge of the genome of different animals grows and increasingly allows us to efficiently identify parts of it that relate to beneficial elements of the phenotype. Of course, the economic cost of such programmes will always be of consequence, especially in the production animal context.

In addition, 'domestication' of more wild species, accelerated by modern genetic knowledge and technologies, is likely to be directed both at adding additional varieties for livestock production and at safeguarding species nearing extinction. Knowledge of the genetic basis of disease and gene therapies is developing rapidly and in future this will be applied widely across species.

In the past, many breeding programmes concentrated on a limited number of parameters because their objectives were often focused on production traits, and computing capability was limited. Modern breeding programmes for livestock can select for many different characteristics concurrently. Modern computing power and specialized programs allow the complex and sensitive analyses needed for this. As already noted, genetics has been and is used to increase the productivity of livestock and poultry and the profitability of different management systems. This emphasis on increased productivity has had negative impacts on some facets of animal welfare, but increasingly included in selection indices are components such as longevity and health (Miglior et al., 2005). Although modern developments in genetics, biotechnology and animal breeding may affect animal welfare positively, monitoring for negative effects will continue to be important.

Part 3

Assessment of Animal Welfare

Animal Welfare, Grading Compromise and Mitigating Suffering

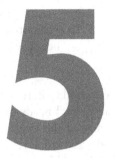

Very good welfare is present when the nutritional, environmental, health, behavioural and mental needs of animals are met fully; that is, when there is no compromise in any of the five domains of welfare (Chapter 1). Very good welfare embodies both very low levels of negative experiences, for example significant hunger, pain, nausea and fear, *and also* the presence of positive experiences, for example satiety, contentment, vitality, enjoyment and playfulness. It is assumed that mammals and birds that can experience, or enjoy, good welfare can also experience its opposite, suffering. Severe suffering, in contrast to good welfare, constitutes deeply unpleasant, undesired states of being which are the outcome of the impact on an animal of a variety of noxious stimuli and/or an absence of important positive stimuli. Clearly there is a range of states between these two extremes. In this chapter, some general features of relationships between degrees of welfare compromise and suffering, how welfare compromise can be graded and general approaches to the mitigation of suffering are considered.

5.1 The Welfare–Suffering Continuum, Good Welfare and Suffering

5.1.1 Animal welfare varies on a continuum of states between very good welfare and severe suffering

The welfare status of an animal at any one time may be envisaged as located on a continuum of states that ranges between very good welfare and severe suffering: the welfare–suffering continuum (Mellor and Reid, 1994). Except at the extremes, an animal's welfare status will be neither completely good nor completely bad. Instead, it will embody a mixture of good, neutral and bad elements resulting physiologically in sensory and other neural inputs that originate in the five domains of welfare. It is the integrated balance and interpretation of all such inputs from the five domains that determine, overall, how positive or negative the animal's perceived experience will be (Chapter 1). Moreover, it is this perceived experience which determines the animal's welfare status and its appropriate location on the welfare–suffering continuum (Figure 5.1). Intermediate welfare states will vary widely in their actual causes and character, and their location on the continuum will be determined by the relative intensities of all the positive and negative inputs and the manner in which these are processed and interpreted by the individual animal experiencing them.

However, this raises a question: how can an animal's welfare status be appropriately located on the welfare–suffering continuum; that is, how can the extent of animal welfare compromise be graded? This question is addressed below, but

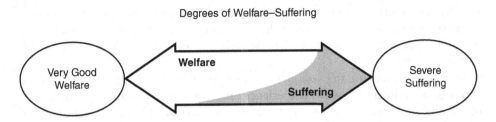

Figure 5.1 The welfare–suffering continuum.

first some other features of relationships between good welfare and suffering are considered.

5.1.2 As welfare decreases suffering increases, and vice versa, but the relationship is complex

In general, it seems obvious that as welfare decreases suffering would increase, and vice versa, so we can recognize that both welfare and suffering have different levels, degrees or intensities. However, the relationship between welfare and suffering is complex for several main reasons (Figure 5.1).

The first, as noted above, is that elements of good welfare may co-exist with elements of reduced or poor welfare. For instance, well-fed, healthy animals in a thermally benign environment may be severely restricted behaviourally, for example caged layer hens and sows in stalls, or well-fed animals kept as a group with more behavioural freedom may be subject to injuries from victimization by others or to microbial infections transmitted from unhygienic deep litter, for example layer hens in barns and group-housed sows.

The second reason is that animals that have a good welfare status because their needs are being met in most of the five domains are likely to tolerate relatively *minor* or even *moderate* compromise in one or more of the domains without the overall experience being strongly negative. One example is a moderate but short-term increase in hunger due to a somewhat extended interval between successive feeds in animals that are otherwise in a good state of welfare. Another example is the quite short-lived but sharp pain of ear tagging in thriving and healthy young animals. Further examples include a mild skin itch caused by lice, mild infection-induced irritation of the air passages of the lungs and mild abdominal discomfort associated with subclinical gastrointestinal infections (bacterial or viral), each occurring in otherwise healthy animals. Likewise, a moderate compromise might be substantially or even entirely mitigated if the animal has feelings of social support, or control over the environment. For example, animals in harmonious social groups respond less fearfully to novel or challenging conditions including movement to new housing and recovery from surgery (De Vries *et al.*, 2003).

Thus, in moving along the continuum from a very good welfare state to where suffering starts to increase, there is likely be a stage before this *tipping point* where the overall experience remains acceptable to the animals because all perceived negative sensations are still tolerable. In other words, high-level welfare can probably deteriorate to some extent without the occurrence of even low-level suffering (Figure 5.1).

The third reason for the complex relationship between welfare and suffering arises because intense negative experiences may be elicited in any one, or more, of the five domains of welfare, and the experiences elicited within each domain may differ. In addition, although those experiences that cause suffering are by definition extremely unpleasant, the negative sensations elicited in one domain may completely dominate those from other domains, or they may be additive or multiplicative. For instance, very severe breathlessness during marked respiratory compromise would probably overwhelm almost any other sensation, whereas nausea and pain may combine in the suffering caused by some severe gastro-intestinal infections. Less severe negative experiences may also impair enjoyment of positive opportunities; for example, animals in barren environments might react to intended enrichments with fear, or animals experiencing even mild pain may withdraw from social contact.

Finally, once the tipping point is reached it is not clear whether suffering increases uniformly, in an accelerating pattern, or in some other pattern, nor whether the pattern of increase depends on the sensory modality involved. Nevertheless, it is clear that suffering can increase from low to exceptionally high levels.

We can potentially integrate these varied experiences onto a single welfare dimension because sentient animals evidently have a perception of their own state and it is this perception that can be understood as ranging from extreme suffering to great satisfaction through a number of intermediate states. Thus, welfare can be seen as ranging in level over a single dimension even though suffering and welfare have separate and distinctive properties where one is not defined solely as the absence of the other, and each arises from an immense number of specific stimuli over time.

5.1.3 Suffering has numerous qualitatively distinct forms: it is not a single entity

There is no single entity of suffering. The word 'suffering' represents a generalized condition of misery resulting from noxious sensory inputs and deficits elicited by significant compromise in one or more of the five domains of welfare. Its dominant form or character depends very much on which sensory modalities are most stimulated and the perceived negative experiences they generate. Examples are provided in Table 5.1. When intense enough, these experiences constitute states of suffering. It is important to note, however, that as each of these forms of suffering becomes more intense and approaches its maximum, the state of suffering induced nevertheless retains its original character. For instance, intense thirst remains thirst, it does not *become* suffering; it simply represents one type of intense negative experience which is described in a generic sense as a state of suffering. Likewise, marked debility, anxiety and the other very unpleasant experiences retain their original forms

Table 5.1 Examples of unpleasant experiences which, at their extreme, represent states of suffering (also see Gregory, 2004).

Column 1: alerting	Column 2: convalescent	Column 3: negative
Thirst	Debility	Loneliness
Hunger	Weakness	Helplessness
Nausea	Sickness	Boredom
Pain (short-lived)	Pain (moderate)	Pain (persistent, untreatable)
Fear	Breathlessness (transient, curable)	Breathlessness (incurable)
Anxiety (transient)	Dizziness	Anxiety (persistent)
Frustration (transient)		Frustration (persistent)
		Distress

and do not *become* suffering, yet they are intense enough for the animal to be described as suffering.

5.1.4 Not all unpleasant experiences that may induce suffering at their extreme are wholly bad

As each of the unpleasant experiences listed in Table 5.1 may lead to suffering at their extreme, it is easy to assume that at any level they are all wholly bad and therefore should be avoided. However, this is an oversimplification. This point is illustrated by assigning these experiences to three broad categories represented by different columns in Table 5.1: *Column 1*, corrective, alerting or protective experiences; *Column 2*, experiences that may promote convalescence; and *Column 3*, negative or destructive experiences. Columns 1 and 2 represent motivating states for action and inaction, respectively. As such they may be functional and necessary for normal behaviours, for example foraging, escape and appeasement, and for learning and a psychologically active life. However, Column 3 represents states that are often chronic and, in addition, cannot be resolved by the animal's own actions. Note that there may be some overlap, so that an experience in one category may be represented in another in a somewhat different form, for example different sorts of pain, curable and incurable breathlessness, and transient and persistent frustration or anxiety.

5.1.4.1 Corrective, alerting or protective experiences

It is obvious that without *thirst* animals will not drink and without *hunger* they will not eat, so that normal daily variations in these experiences tend to promote animal welfare. *Nausea* can be protective in two main ways: first, it is often accompanied by vomiting, which helps animals to rid themselves of the ingested feed that contains the potentially hazardous chemicals or microbial agents that cause the nausea; and second, in associating nausea with particular feeds, the animal may learn to avoid those feeds in the future. *Pain,* usually short-lived pain, alerts animals to potential or actual tissue damage. It then elicits protective movement away from the injurious stimulus, causes the animal to seek aid from others, and/or induces learning so that the pain-causing situation may be avoided in future. *Fear* also has protective functions in that it may enhance rapid escape or defence responses when animals are unexpectedly confronted by danger, or it may, by eliciting caution, lead animals to avoid potentially dangerous situations, for example unfamiliar environments or proximity to animals perceived as threatening. Transient *frustration* and *anxiety* may occur when animals suspect that their behaviour will not influence whether or not they will receive rewards or punishments.

Clearly, without the negative quality of all of these usually transient experiences and the responses they elicit, the animals would be disadvantaged. To this extent, therefore, their negative quality acts to promote animal welfare. In reacting to these stimuli, some animals perform behaviours such as foraging that give access to emotional satisfaction, activity, learning and a sense of control over their environment. Also, stimuli that provoke huddling, burrowing and nest building in rodents may lead to greater welfare than would providing a constant, thermally neutral environment which suppresses these behaviours and leaves the animal unoccupied. In fact, some behaviours, such as play, may function partly to bring about transient surprise and loss of control and thereby improve the animal's ability to recover from them (Spinka *et al.*, 2001).

5.1.4.2 Experiences that may promote convalescence

Debility, *weakness* and *sickness* are generally disabling and induce a behavioural response of inactivity. Affected animals may sleep, and often isolate themselves from others (Gregory, 1998). Lingering but transient moderate *pain* can have rather similar effects (Mellor *et al.*, 2000), as can *dizziness*. The induced immobility may aid convalescence. If the cause is invading microorganisms, immobility reduces the use of energy for muscular contractions and thereby makes more energy available for mounting body immune defence responses. The same is true for the energy-expensive inflammatory and repair processes that follow tissue damage due to, for instance, traumatic injury, surgical intervention, burns and poisons, as well as damaging microorganisms. Likewise, immobility or reduced mobility due to *breathlessness* minimises the consumption of oxygen when its supply is limited. This helps to safeguard brain function and thereby would have convalescent benefits provided that the cause of the breathlessness is reversible, for example transiently impaired lung function during an infection, and curable heart disease. Although these experiences do not encourage behaviourally active solutions, they are still functional because the animal can exercise a degree of control by reducing them through inactivity.

5.1.4.3 Negative or destructive experiences

A major feature of the negative experiences in this category (Column 3) that distinguishes them from those in the other two (Columns 1 and 2) is that, in general, they do not appear to elicit behavioural or physiological responses that can act to improve animal welfare. In effect, in these cases what the animal does cannot allow it to substantially resolve or escape the aversive stimuli and it enters a chronic state of suffering. Category 3 experiences include different forms of welfare compromise over the full range of negative impacts from quite low to very high. Five of these negative emotional states – *loneliness/depression, helplessness, boredom, chronic anxiety* and *frustration* – largely arise through the impact on the animal of its long-term housing environment. In domesticated circumstances, therefore, human intervention is required to reduce or eliminate these experiences. *Distress,* as a strongly negative, predominantly emotional experience falls into a similar category, but it might also accompany the combined physical and emotional experiences of unremitting *pain* or persistent severely disabling *breathlessness*. In those cases, relief of the symptoms would require therapeutic intervention, but if the pain is untreatable or the cause of breathlessness is incurable, euthanasia may be needed to relieve suffering that is severe enough to undermine the animal's enjoyment of life.

5.1.5 An absence of positive experiences, as distinct from the presence of negative ones, may also compromise animal welfare

Up to this point the focus has been on the presence of emphatically negative states, largely because animal welfare science to date has, with few exceptions, only embraced notions of severe welfare compromise caused by explicitly noxious inputs. As noted in Chapter 1, however, other forms of welfare compromise may be related to an absence of positive mental states; for instance, those related to feelings of reward or satisfaction. Thus, such compromise may occur in circumstances which hinder an animal's capacity to experience such things as vitality, companionship, contentment, satiety, happiness, curiosity, exploration, foraging and play. Indeed, it has been suggested in animal psychology, as also in human psychology, that a good life comes from the presence of positive experiences (Koene and Duncan, 2001) and diffuse as well as specifically motivated feelings (Wemelsfelder, 1997a). Perhaps the explicitly negative causes of suffering are currently too plentiful and urgent, so that researchers are understandably in 'rescue' mode and unable to step back and consider, more widely, the features of a good life. Or perhaps the complex and holistic nature of the task is, as yet, too daunting. Whatever the answer, while noting this as a developing area of interest, the following discussion emphasizes explicitly negative states and allows for the possibility that the deprivation of opportunities for positive experience, once convincingly established as a significant form of welfare compromise, could be included in the grading system enumerated below.

5.1.6 Recognition of suffering in animals is mainly by analogy with human experience

As suffering is a subjective state perceived by the animal, recognizing suffering in animals inevitably requires us to interpret their behavioural and functional states using human experience as our reference point (Gregory, 2004). This is because we cannot understand the unpleasantness of states involving breathlessness, nausea, pain and so on, in any other way (Table 5.1). However, although a degree of similarity may be anticipated, caution is needed because such animal and human experiences are not necessarily the same – that is, not identical – and not all higher animals may experience all such states. Indeed, there is evidence that the dynamics, character and significance of sensory inputs that underlie experiences that are sufficiently noxious to cause suffering may differ between animals and human beings. For instance, there are well-known differences in the capabilities of some sensory modalities, for example much greater olfactory sensitivity in dogs, auditory range in rats and visual acuity in raptors than in human beings, and some animals possess unique sensory modalities, for example echolocation in cetaceans and sonar in bats.

Nevertheless, carefully considered human-to-animal extrapolations may be undertaken in cases where sensory modalities are common to both and where behavioural and functional parameters also suggest strong parallels. This is especially so where it would be generally assumed that, with few exceptions, particular sensory experiences are similar across mammalian and possibly avian species. For instance, high-level thirst and hunger, pain, fear, sickness and breathlessness would probably fall into this category. Indeed, it may be possible to assess this as operant studies allow the strength of aversions produced by basic experiences, such as hunger, to be compared to more species-specific experiences. However, it is not necessary to show that the nature of such shared noxious experiences is precisely the same in animals and human beings for us to give due weight to the potential for animals to suffer. It is only necessary to adopt the ethical position that unpleasant experiences such as these, which have a character, intensity and duration that are sufficient to cause suffering, are as significant to the animal in its terms as these experiences are to us in our human terms.

5.2 Grading Animal Welfare Compromise

5.2.1 Grading welfare compromise is important in many contexts
Animal welfare status needs to be monitored in all circumstances where animals are used for human purposes. These circumstances vary widely and involve many different species (Table 5.2). In some cases, we would expect monitoring to reassure us that the animals are faring well and that no action is required. In others, we would expect compromised welfare to be demonstrated, thereby indicating a need to take remedial action. We might also expect that when the demands we place on animals require them to operate close to the limits of their behavioural or functional capacities the more likely it is that their welfare will be compromised. Moreover, if such compromise were severe enough the animals would suffer. Whatever the situation, we need the capacity to assess the nature and degree of welfare compromise,

Table 5.2 Use of sentient animals for human purposes (adapted from Spedding, 2000).

Category of animals	Examples of species used
Farm	Cattle, goats, sheep, deer, buffaloes, camels, alpacas, pigs, horses, donkeys, poultry, emus, ostriches, monkeys
Work	Bullocks, buffaloes, horses, donkeys, mules, dogs, elephants, llamas, ferrets, cormorants
Sport	Horses, dogs, camels, bulls, steers, calves, pigs, hawks, pigeons, pheasants, whales; *hunting*: dogs, hawks, horses; *hunted*: deer, pigs, rabbits, foxes, big game, game birds
Companion	Dogs, cats, ponies, donkeys, rabbits, rats, mice, hamsters, birds, reptiles, amphibians
Captive	Large cats, elephants, giraffes, monkeys, bears, otters, range ruminants, birds, reptiles, amphibians
Wild	Foxes, rabbits, deer, pigs, large cats, game birds
Those used in science	Rabbits, rats, mice, monkeys, dogs, cats, all farmed ruminants, pigs, horses, reptiles, amphibians, fish

however severe it is. This is fundamental to promoting and maintaining good welfare, to identifying poor welfare, and to gauging the effectiveness of actions designed to correct welfare compromise. In addition, the features of the animal's environment and the attributes of all management procedures employed should be proactively assessed and, where possible, changed to expose animals to lower risks of welfare compromise.

On one level, welfare cannot be directly measured or reliably known, yet in applied settings is must be assessed in very specific terms to determine whether the animal's status is acceptable, and to direct attempts at amelioration when it is judged to be compromised. The following grading scheme provides a structure for examining animal welfare in all contexts of human use. For illustrative purposes farm animals and animals used in science will be considered. In both categories, significant, sometimes very marked, welfare impositions are placed on some animals.

5.2.1.1 Farm animals
The nature and degree of welfare compromise in farm livestock may differ with the species (e.g. dairy cattle, sheep, layer hens), the farming purpose (e.g. meat, milk, eggs, fibre), the management system (e.g. pasture-based, feed-lot, fully housed), the management procedure (e.g. gathering, marking, transporting, slaughtering), the life stage of the animal (e.g. newborn, growing, mature, pregnant, lactating), the farming environment (e.g. arid/verdant, alpine/tundra/savannah) and the climate (e.g. frigid, temperate, torrid). Having access to a grading system that would aid welfare assessments in this wide range of contexts would therefore be most helpful.

This is perhaps especially important with commercial animals used on farms, because the need to remain financially viable commonly requires some animal welfare trade-offs (Mellor and Stafford, 2001), and this may mean that the animals are managed close to the margin between acceptable and unacceptable welfare. Thus, effective management of farm livestock would be facilitated by the ability to distinguish between acceptable and unacceptable welfare states and to grade and respond appropriately to the welfare compromises that may occur at our hands.

5.2.1.2 Animals used in science: research, teaching and testing

Scientific uses of animals that cause them harm may be justified ethically only when the anticipated benefits substantially outweigh the negative impact on the animals *and* when all practicable measures have been taken to minimize any harm (Mellor and Reid, 1994; Mellor, 1998). Societal support for such use of animals depends critically on scientists fulfilling both obligations. A capacity to assess the welfare status and to grade the nature and degree of any welfare compromise caused by scientific investigations is central to this. This requires a grading system that is versatile and comprehensive enough to cover the wide range of procedures deployed in the many animal species used (Table 5.2), and the numerous forms of welfare compromise that may occur. Such a system was devised by Mellor and Reid (1994), and since 1997 has been part of the regulatory framework for managing the scientific use of animals in New Zealand (Williams *et al.*, 2006) and elsewhere.

5.2.2 A system for grading animal welfare comprehensively is available

The original system devised by Mellor and Reid (1994) relied heavily on the then novel concept of the five domains of potential welfare compromise. The value of these domains in illuminating animal welfare thinking and practice beyond its initial focus on the use of animals in science soon became evident. Accordingly, with some modification in the intervening period (Mellor and Stafford, 2001) the five domains and their interactions (Figure 5.2) have now become important facets of our animal welfare thinking, with relevance to all areas of animal use, as indicated in this book. This points to the potential to use the related grading system, somewhat modified, more widely than was originally envisaged. A major advantage is the comprehensiveness of the system because, in resting on the five domains, it is hard to envisage any welfare insult that would not be captured within one or more of the domains. The system has the following additional key attributes.

5.2.2.1 The nature of welfare compromise is assessed

The system allows the *nature* of welfare compromise to be assessed thoroughly by reference to the five domains (Figure 5.2). Careful evaluation of an animal's status in each domain allows the potential impact of sensory and other neural inputs from each of the first four broadly physical domains to be assessed in terms of their possible contributions to the animal's experience in the fifth,

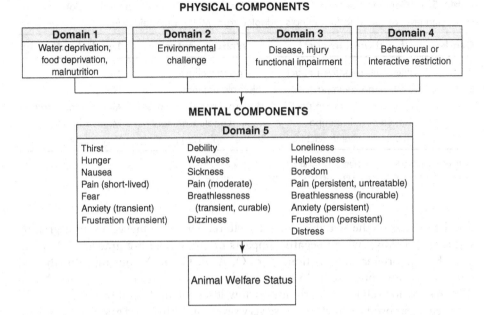

PHYSICAL COMPONENTS

Domain 1	Domain 2	Domain 3	Domain 4
Water deprivation, food deprivation, malnutrition	Environmental challenge	Disease, injury functional impairment	Behavioural or interactive restriction

MENTAL COMPONENTS

Domain 5

Thirst	Debility	Loneliness
Hunger	Weakness	Helplessness
Nausea	Sickness	Boredom
Pain (short-lived)	Pain (moderate)	Pain (persistent, untreatable)
Fear	Breathlessness	Breathlessness (incurable)
Anxiety (transient)	(transient, curable)	Anxiety (persistent)
Frustration (transient)	Dizziness	Frustration (persistent)
		Distress

Animal Welfare Status

Figure 5.2 Domains of potential welfare compromise divided broadly into physical and mental components. Modified from Mellor and Reid (1994) and Mellor (2004a).

mental domain. Examples are water deprivation leading to thirst, inflammation of the upper respiratory passages leading to soreness and irritation, a collapsed lung or pneumonia to breathlessness, septicaemia (blood poisoning) to sickness, lacerations to pain, and so on. Also, direct consideration of the mental domain itself allows evaluation of inputs that are largely independent of the other four domains, for example inputs such as those linked to a perceived threat manifesting as fear. As already noted (Table 5.1), these are just some of numerous examples of unpleasant, sometimes noxious, experiences that an animal may have.

5.2.2.2 Grades are determined by impacts on function

The grades are differentiated by reference to the general functional capacities of the animals. Thus, distinctions are made on the basis of the following three factors: (1) the severity of functional disruption, (2) the duration of the disruption and its reversibility and (3) whether or not the noxious effects might need to be mitigated or ended by relocation to more benign conditions, by therapeutic intervention and/or by euthanasia. On this basis, the grades represent increasingly negative impacts on the animals, impacts that will be likely to impair welfare or, at the extreme, cause suffering. These impacts may be described in general terms (Table 5.3) or in more

Table 5.3 General description of grades on the functional impact scale, the related welfare status and level of suffering for animals (adapted from Mellor and Reid, 1994).

Grade	Functional impact[a]	Welfare status[b]	Level of suffering[b]
A	Little or no negative impact	Very good welfare	None
B	Minor negative impact	Tolerable unpleasantness	None
C	Moderate negative impact	Moderate unpleasantness	Minor to moderate
D	Marked negative impact	Marked unpleasantness	Marked to severe
E	Severe negative impact	Severe unpleasantness	Very severe

[a]Relates to the degree of functional disruptions (Domains 1–4).
[b]Relates to the negative mental experience of the animal (Domain 5).

detail for each of the five domains of welfare. This is achieved using a grading system (see below), where negative impacts on an animal are graded as A, B, C, D or E (The original designations were O, A, B, C and X, but this alphabetical sequence is now preferred). In terms of the animal's experience, grades A and B represent no welfare compromise to low-level tolerable compromise, grade E represents compromise likely to cause very severe suffering, and grades C and D are intermediate levels (Table 5.3).

5.2.2.3 The degree of welfare compromise is graded
The system allows the *degree* or *intensity* of compromise to be gauged. As before, each domain is assessed in turn and the integrated outcome in the mental domain is graded according to the anticipated *intensity* of the negative feelings. This is done using the five-point impact scale (A–E) applied to all five domains.

Designating the steps numerically from 1 to 5 has been explicitly rejected in order to prevent glib, unreflective averaging of 'scores' as a substitute for considered judgement (Mellor and Reid, 1994; Williams *et al.*, 2006). Judgement is required because, as we have already seen (Chapter 1), the relative noxiousness of the different unpleasant experiences animals (or human beings) may have is very difficult to gauge. For instance, how can one compare the different experiences of breathlessness, nausea and pain? Likewise, although the relative intensities of one or a particular combination of these unpleasant experiences can often be graded, for example pain alone or pain plus nausea, the impact of contributions from within the four physical domains on the intensity of the experience in the mental domain is not always clear.

5.2.3 The grading system employs stratified impact assessments in all five welfare domains
The impact at each grade for each of the five domains of welfare is outlined in more detail here, and some examples are given in Table 5.4.

Table 5.4 Examples of indices of functional disruption in the five domains of welfare (e.g. Morton and Griffiths, 1985; Blood and Radostits, 1989; Mellor et al., 2000; Aitken, 2007).

Domain	Disruption	Indices
1 Nutrition	Dehydration	Skin 'tenting', ↑ blood cell and protein levels, ↓ blood and urine water content; ↓ urine output
	Undernutrition	↓ Body condition score, ↓ or ↑ in blood levels of metabolites
	Malnutrition	Clinical or subclinical indices of deficiency or excess
2 Environment	Cold exposure	Shivering, ↓ body temperature, ↑ heat production
	Heat exposure	Sweating/panting, ↑ body temperature, seeking shade
3 Health	Disease	Fever, ↑ heart rate, inflammation of mucous membranes, mucus from body orifices, lung congestion, vomiting, diarrhoea, and numerous other pathogen-specific, toxin-specific, genetic and other symptoms or indices
	Injuries	Visible cuts, bruises, abrasions, fractures; torn ligaments and tendons; organ ruptures; bleeding; burns, scalds, inflamed tissues; posture; demeanour; mobility; vocalization
4 Behaviour	Restrictions	Absence of, e.g. normal reproductive, nest-building, locomotor, foraging, territory inspection/marking, hunting, social or solitary, vocal and other behaviours
		Presence of behavioural vices or damaging or otherwise abnormal behaviours, e.g. self-mutilation or self-injuring, stereotyped (aimlessly repetitive actions), withdrawn, anxious, fearful, aggressive or other such behaviours
5 Mental	Thirst, hunger	Responses to water and food
	Breathlessness	Breathing (depth, rate, sound), blue colour of mouth membranes, inability to perform even mild exercise
	Anxiety, fear, pain, distress	*Physiological indices*, e.g. ↑ stress hormone levels and related metabolites, ↑ heart rate, altered breathing (rate and depth), ↑ body temperature, ↑ sweating, ↑ red blood cell levels, ↓ immune defences, muscle tremor
		Behaviour, e.g. numerous different forms of vocalisation, posture, locomotion and temperament, specific to the problem and species
	Nausea, sickness, debility, weakness	Mainly behaviour and demeanour

5.2.3.1 Domain 1 Nutrition: water deprivation, food deprivation, malnutrition

Grade A

Water/fluid is available in quantities which avoid dehydration. Food of appropriate types and compositions for the species is available in amounts which meet body maintenance requirements plus any additional demands imposed by factors such as pregnancy, lactation, growth, exercise, thermal challenge or recuperation from illness or injury.

Grade B

Water/fluid or food restrictions or excesses cause minor, readily reversible effects on physiological state, body condition or performance.

Grade C

Water/fluid or food restrictions or excesses cause serious short-term or moderate long-term effects on physiological state, body condition or performance, but such effects remain within the capacity of the body to respond to nutritional variations and allow spontaneous recovery after the restoration of a good-quality diet at the required intake.

Grade D

Water/fluid or food restrictions or excesses lead to levels of debility where euthanasia would be used to avoid an inevitable further decline because therapy would either be ineffective or too protracted.

Grade E

Water/fluid or food restrictions or excesses result in a predicted end point of death.

5.2.3.2 Domain 2 Environment: challenging outdoor and indoor conditions

Grade A

Outdoor or indoor environmental conditions elicit body responses that remain within the animal's capacity to react to external stimuli without recourse to adaptive physiological changes, for example no change in heat production.

Grade B

Environmental conditions cause body responses that remain within the normal wider capacity of the animals to react to, but they involve adaptive physiological responses, for example an increase in heat production.

Grade C

Environmental conditions represent marked short-term or moderate long-term environmental challenges that elicit body responses beyond the physiological adaptive capacity of the animals, but the untoward effects are readily reversed by restoration of benign conditions with or without additional therapeutic intervention.

Grade D
Environmental conditions represent extreme environmental challenges that lead to serious physiological compromise, where euthanasia would be used to prevent an inevitable further decline or because therapeutic procedures would be ineffective or too protracted.

Grade E
Environmental conditions cause protracted extreme physiological compromise or the end point is death.

5.2.3.3 Domain 3 Health: disease, injury, functional impairment
Grade A
Good health with no significant disease, injury or functional impairment.

Grade B
Health challenges cause body responses that remain within the normal wider capacity of the animals to react to with no or only minor debility or incapacity.

Grade C
Health challenges cause marked short-term or moderate long-term functional changes associated with moderate debility or incapacity, but from which complete recovery occurs spontaneously or can be readily achieved therapeutically.

Grade D
Health challenges cause marked debility or incapacity and serious physiological compromise, where euthanasia would be used to prevent an inevitable further decline because therapeutic procedures would be ineffective or too protracted. Health challenges cause death unpredictably in a small proportion of animals because a rapid deterioration in their state can occur with little or no warning.

Grade E
Health challenges in conscious animals cause extreme debility or incapacity or the predicted end point is an unpleasant death.

5.2.3.4 Domain 4 Behaviour: individual, group or interactive restrictions
Grade A
Restrictions do not interfere with the behavioural needs of individuals or groups of animals (an animal's behavioural needs being those activities which when thwarted produce untoward physiological or psychological effects).

Grade B
Restrictions cause minor interference with the satisfaction of behavioural needs of individuals or groups of animals.

Grade C
Restrictions cause marked short-term or moderate long-term interference with the satisfactions of behavioural needs of individuals or groups of animals, leading

to untoward physiological or psychological effects which are readily reversed by the restoration of benign conditions with or without additional therapeutic intervention.

Grade D
Restrictions markedly interfere with the satisfactions of behavioural needs of individuals or groups of animals leading to severe physiological or psychological compromise requiring restoration of benign conditions, with or without additional therapeutic intervention, or the use of euthanasia to limit the magnitude or duration, or both, of the imposed compromise.

Grade E
Circumstances cause severe interference with the satisfactions of the behavioural needs of individuals or groups of animals, leading to psychotic-like behaviour or to agonistic interactions that result in severe injury or death.

5.2.3.5 Domain 5 Mental state: unpleasant or noxious experiences
Grade A
Benign circumstances do not lead to any unpleasant experiences.

Grade B
Circumstances in which any unpleasant experiences occur at tolerable low levels.

Grade C
Circumstances in which unpleasant experiences occur at moderate levels for short periods or at low levels for long periods.

Grade D
Circumstances in which unpleasant or noxious experiences are marked, where any suffering caused is ended by euthanasia or by therapeutic or other interventions before it becomes excessive, or where the suffering is short-lived and complete recovery can occur. Circumstances in which unpleasant experiences occur at moderate levels for long periods.

Grade E
Circumstances lead to severe, inescapable or unrelieved noxious experiences where the intensity or duration, or both, of the induced suffering are at or beyond the limits of reasonable endurance.

5.2.4 There are specific indices for assessing functional compromise in the five domains
The general characterization of the grades in each domain just described has its foundation in the accumulated knowledge of functional disruptions studied by numerous scientists, veterinarians and others over at least the last 50 years (Mellor and Bayvel, 2008). Although such grading of compromise probably had not been systematized to this extent before 1994 (Mellor and Reid, 1994), judgements of

this character were nevertheless made, perhaps especially by veterinarians and animal-based scientists (e.g. Morton and Griffiths, 1985; Blood and Radostits, 1989; Mellor and Bayvel, 2008) as part of their daily engagement with animals in clinical, production and scientific contexts. Accordingly, there are numerous useful indices already available within the veterinary clinical arena, as well as in applied nutritional, environmental, behavioural and neural/cognitive spheres, which can now be deployed to support systematic animal welfare assessments. Indeed, there are so many that listing all of them here is impractical, and only a few examples are provided in Table 5.4. It is important to note, however, that such indices relate to the degree of functional disruption in each of the domains; what such disruptions mean in terms of the likely experience the animals may have requires the careful exercise of informed judgement (see Chapter 1).

5.2.5 Overall welfare status depends on the accumulated grade in the mental domain

5.2.5.1 General use of the system

When undertaking a detailed assessment using the grading system, animals in each situation must be graded in all five domains of potential welfare compromise. The overall grading would usually be that assigned to Domain 5, mental state (Figure 5.2). However, grading in all five domains is necessary to help ensure that all factors that may contribute to welfare compromise of different kinds are assessed. When assessing compromise in each domain care must be taken to avoid inclusion of those compromises dealt with in the other domains. The greatest anticipated compromise specific to each domain should be used when assigning the grade within each domain. When compromise in two or more domains is anticipated to contribute to an animal's negative experience, assigning an appropriately higher grade to Domain 5 should be considered. If the grade in Domain 5 is not known, the highest grade in Domains 1–4 should probably be taken as the overall grade.

The emphasis here is on the welfare status of the animal, the *welfare output*, not on the *management and resource inputs* that achieve it. Detailed welfare grading of this sort described here may be more readily applicable to individuals or to small groups of animals than to large numbers and, in addition, could be particularly useful when evidence is being gathered to support or defend prosecutions for mistreatment of animals. Nevertheless, such insights into the negative mental experiences animals may have are essential components of welfare assessments of large groups, especially in the context of on-farm assurance schemes. The Bristol Welfare Assurance Programme is a particularly good example (Webster, 2005a). It has three key components: first, *an assessment of the welfare status* of the animals using behaviour, demeanour, appearance, physiological and clinical state, and so on; second, *an evaluation of management inputs* in terms of the procedures in place to care for the animals and, closely allied to these, the quality and empathy of the stockmanship; and third, *the resources deployed* in terms of food quality and availability and the standard, upkeep and suitability of the facilities including accommodation, yards, races and so on. Strengths of this programme include the capacity to assess the present welfare status of the animals and how management and resource factors contribute to that status, and the capacity to correct current problems and anticipate and thereby avoid or minimize future problems.

5.2.5.2 Grading scientific procedures

The ethical responsibilities of scientists to fully assess the potential negative impacts of their procedures on the animals they study (Mellor, 1998) demand the use of a detailed and comprehensive grading system which allows the animal's likely mental state to be gauged (Mellor and Reid, 1994). The process of determining the overall grade in such studies is illustrated by the five examples in Table 5.5. They show that all domains are considered and that, with few exceptions, the grade assigned to mental state is the chief determinant of the overall grade. The first three examples show that the overall grade is the same as that assigned to Domain 5. In the fourth example the grade in Domain 5 is greater than any of the individual grades because compromise in two other domains is anticipated to magnify the negative experience. The last example shows that in the absence of compromise to mental state, graded A in Domain 5, the highest grade in one of the other domains becomes the overall grade.

Each experimental group in a scientific study needs to be graded separately, to ensure that the grade assigned to animals receiving the most severe treatment, for example induction of a debilitating disease, is not assigned to groups which are treated more benignly, for example non-diseased control groups. This helps to ensure that the severity of compromise imposed on all animals in an experiment is neither under- nor overestimated (Williams *et al.*, 2006). Note should be made of ratings given to similar procedures by different individuals and institutions to ensure that appropriate and transparent assessments of the animal's status are being undertaken, especially as there are extra restrictions and regulatory burdens associated with judging an animal's welfare to be moderately or severely compromised.

Mellor and Reid (1994) provided examples of the grading assigned in each domain for a wide range of scientific procedures. Some of these are illustrated here for Domain 5, the mental state (Table 5.6).

5.3 Mitigation of Suffering

The following points should now be apparent. First, suffering is a generalized condition of misery resulting from noxious sensory inputs or deficits elicited by significant compromise in one or more of the five domains of welfare (Figure 5.2). Second, the character of suffering (Table 5.1) depends on which sensory modality or modalities dominate in determining the nature of an animal's unpleasant mental experience. Third, the sensory modalities that dominate are determined largely by the welfare domain(s) in which compromise occurs. Fourth, welfare compromise

Table 5.5 Examples of grading the overall impact of animal welfare compromise during five scientific studies (adapted from Mellor and Reid, 1994). In each case, the impact is graded in the five domains of potential welfare compromise and an overall grade is assigned.

Domain	Description of impact	Grade
Study 1: Limited gut resection (removal) and its consequences		
1	Fluid/food intake affected slightly	B
2	Thermoneutral environment	A
3	Anaesthesia plus surgery with effective analgesia	C
4	Minor behavioural restriction (indoor individual pen)	B
5	Moderate pain/distress (mainly with surgery)	C
		Overall: C
Study 2: Blood sampling of recently confined and untamed free-range domesticated animals with strong flight responses		
1	Fluid/food intake affected slightly (reduced for first 48 h)	B
2	Thermoneutral environment	A
3	Simple venepuncture of healthy uninjured animals	B
4	Mild behavioural restriction (handling, large indoor pen)	B
5	Marked fear/distress (mainly from handling/restraint)	D
		Overall: D
Study 3: Usually fatal viral diarrhoea in hand-reared newborn animals		
1	Fluid/food intake moderately affected	C
2	Thermoneutral environment	A
3	Extreme debility or functional compromise	E
4	Minor behavioural restriction	B
5	Severe pain/distress (mainly from gut effects)	E
		Overall: E
Study 4: Underfed animals exposed to severe cold for a short period (24 h)		
1	Food intake restricted to cause weight loss of 20%	C
2	Cold challenge at the limit of the animal's adaptive response	C
3	Mild functional impairment	B
4	Mild behavioural restriction (indoor individual pen)	B
5	Marked overall distress (from underfeeding and cold)	D
		Overall: D
Study 5: Operant conditioning with positive reinforcement using animals accustomed to the experimental environment and apparatus		
1	Fluid/food intake unaffected	A
2	Thermoneutral environment	A
3	Healthy, uninjured animals	A
4	Minor behavioural restriction	B
5	No significant negative experience	A
		Overall: A

Table 5.6 Examples of grading for mental state (Domain 5, mental state: unpleasant or noxious experience) for a range of scientific procedures[a] (adapted from Mellor and Reid, 1994).

Grade	Mental state: unpleasant or noxious experiences
A	*Studies which do not lead to any unpleasant experiences*
	For instance field observations of grazing behaviour on farms; studies in thermally or barometrically neutral conditions; benign handling of tamed and trained animals which are familiar with all personnel and procedures and with the place where the procedures are conducted.
B	*Studies in which any unpleasant experiences occur at low levels*
	For instance short-term overall food-intake restrictions, short-term mild cold or heat exposure, studies on completely anaesthetized animals which do not regain consciousness, standard methods of euthanasia that rapidly induce unconsciousness (e.g. anaesthetic overdose), simple venepuncture or venesection, injection of non-toxic substances, skin tests which cause low-level irritation without ulceration, feeding trained animals by orogastric tube, movement of free-range domesticated animals to unfamiliar housing.
C	*Studies in which unpleasant experiences occur at moderate levels for short periods or at low levels for long periods*
	For instance dietary induction of mild deficiency or toxicity symptoms; short-term exposure to severe cold or heat which would lead to collapse if prolonged; induction of mild reversible infectious diarrhoea; recovery from major surgeries such as thorocotomy, orthopaedic procedures, hysterectomy or gall bladder removal, with effective use of anaesthetics during surgery and analgesics afterwards; surgical procedures on conscious animals but with the use of local anaesthesia and systemic analgesic; movement of excitable free-range domesticated livestock to unfamiliar housing.

D   *Studies in which unpleasant or noxious experiences are marked, where any suffering caused is ended by euthanasia or by therapeutic or other interventions before it becomes excessive, or where the suffering is short-lived and complete recovery can occur; studies in which unpleasant experiences occur at moderate levels for long periods*

For instance studies of severe deleterious effects of dietary toxins; prolonged exposure to severe cold which would lead to failure of thermoregulation and collapse, but the exposure is terminated just before those outcomes; induction of severe diarrhoea or severe infectious pneumonia; recovery from major surgery under anaesthesia without the use of analgesics; marked social or environmental deprivation; capture, handling, restraint or housing, without the use of tranquillisers, of wild or semi-domesticated animals that exhibit marked flight responses.

E   *Studies which lead to severe, inescapable or unrelieved noxious experiences where the intensity or duration, or both, of the induced suffering are at or beyond the limits of reasonable endurance*

For instance severe water/fluid or feed restrictions leading to extreme debility or death; exposure to lethal extremes of cold, heat or barometric pressure; evaluation of vaccines where death is the measure of failure to protect; conducting major surgeries without the use of anaesthesia (e.g. where the animal is immobilized physically or with muscle relaxants); testing the efficacy of analgesics in conscious animals with induced severe pain; studies which cause profound withdrawal, agitation, self-mutilation or aggression towards others.

ᵃOutcomes of studies with primary effects in the first four domains usually contribute to the grading in the fifth domain.

is due mainly to the effects of external factors and the functional disruptions they cause. Fifth, the ultimate impact is on the internal mental state the animal experiences (Figure 5.2). It follows that suffering can be mitigated by managing the *external factors*, by treating the associated *functional disruptions* that lead to noxious sensory inputs, and/or by direct treatment of the animal's *mental state*.

5.3.1 Managing external factors that impact on animals can avoid or mitigate suffering

Clearly, avoiding suffering altogether is preferable to mitigating it when it arises, and that is the obvious primary objective of virtually all codes of practice for managing animals. Giving proper attention to the practical management of the animal's nutrition, environment, health, behavioural expression and mental state will pre-empt untoward welfare effects in these domains. How this may be achieved has already been outlined in general terms (see details of grades A and B in each domain). In brief, avoidance of suffering requires the provision of physical resources such as appropriate feed and accommodation or shelter, hygienic conditions, opportunities for functional behavioural expression, and suitable handling facilities, all of which must be managed appropriately (Webster, 2005a), and, of equal importance, it also requires the involvement of empathetic, knowledgeable and skilled animal-handling staff (Webster, 2005a; Chapter 7).

It follows that when suffering occurs, the most direct avenue for mitigating it, and certainly an area that requires attention, is to identify and if possible correct any detrimentally misaligned external factors. In some cases, merely correcting the offending external factors will be sufficient. For instance, an iodine deficiency sufficient to cause weakness may be able to be corrected by a dietary adjustment without the need to inject iodine systemically. Likewise, hypothermia which leads to weakness and debility in newborn lambs, kids and bovine calves immediately after birth may be corrected by simply placing them in warm air, although a mitigating effect of dulled consciousness during hypothermia may complicate assessments of suffering in these circumstances (Mellor and Stafford, 2004). Belly nosing in young pigs typically results when rooting materials are not supplied, and is avoided by addressing this deficiency. Finally, mental states that are less substrate-specific, including helplessness, isolation, boredom or frustration (Table 5.1) caused by barren and/or restricted environments, may be treated by deploying enrichment strategies or by transferring animals to more varied environments (Chapter 8). However, environmental deficits early in life may cause lasting changes in the animal so that their behaviour remains malfunctional even after the deficit has been corrected.

5.3.2 Treating externally caused functional disruptions can reduce noxious sensory inputs that cause suffering

When external factors cause functional disruptions that are severe enough to require therapeutic interventions because those disruptions cannot be corrected by adjusting the external factors, those factors nevertheless require appropriate modification.

The purpose is to protect other animals in the same circumstances that may not yet be affected, and to provide suitable conditions for affected animals when they are returned after being treated successfully. For instance, poor hygiene in dairy calf-rearing units can lead to severe bacterial diarrhoea that requires antibiotic treatment because improving the hygiene alone will not save the affected calves. Also, exhibit animals (e.g. in zoos) with fixed stereotypies may show little response to enriched housing, but such enrichment may prevent the development of this behaviour in others in the group. A final example is where poorly designed or constructed flooring leads to serious limb injuries, such as fractures, which require direct treatment because, obviously, repairing the floor does not mend broken bones. In all three examples, successful treatment would resolve the associated unpleasant experiences of weakness, debility, pain or distress. Note, however, that focusing only on the functional disruption without treating the associated unpleasant mental effects could result in protracted suffering. For example, merely realigning and pinning badly fractured bones under general anaesthesia would usually help to restore the functional integrity of the bones, but post-operative pain would probably persist for some days unless analgesics were also given.

5.3.3 Treating an animal's mental state directly can mitigate suffering

The remaining strategy is to treat the negative mental states directly. There would be strong impetus to do so when the intensities or durations of these mental states were beyond those required to elicit a beneficial reactive response from the animal (Figure 5.1, Column 1) or to promote convalescence (Column 2), and when their continued presence was of no apparent benefit (Column 3). A number of analgesics that target different parts of pain nerve pathways and brain processing areas are available for use with acute (short-lived) pain, but chronic (long-term) pain and its management in animals are not yet well understood (Flecknell and Waterman-Pearson, 2000; Mellor and Stafford, 2000; Stafford and Mellor, 2005a, 2005b; Mellor *et al.*, 2008b). Anti-nausea and anti-dizziness drugs are available for human use, but at present are seldom used in animals. Their correct use would depend very much on the precise causes of nausea and/or dizziness, which would be quite difficult to determine in animals. Anxiolytic drugs have been demonstrated to bind to appropriate receptors in the brain of some animals, and therefore might have a use in animals experiencing apparent feelings of fear, anxiety, helplessness, isolation, boredom and frustration which persist after environmental enrichment and other such strategies have been employed (Chapter 8).

5.3.4 Promoting positive experiences, as distinct from correcting negative ones, may also help to mitigate suffering

Certain behaviours such as play and 'laughter' vocalizations, as identified in rats and dogs, might represent 'sentinels' of happiness amenable to empirical measurement. However, like sentinels of suffering, such as behavioural stereotypy, their causes are likely to be more complex than we currently appreciate. Indeed, the two are likely to be related as, unlike the use of mechanical equipment in agriculture and science, animals are not mere machines which cease to function when we are not using them directly. Rather, their physiological and psychological apparatus is always running and always requires both the absence of destructive inputs (see above) and, importantly, the presence of constructive ones, including occupation which is meaningful to them. Thus, rather than dealing mainly with the negative (suffering) and letting the positive (welfare) look after itself, in many cases it may be more effective to do the reverse. For instance, if animals are provided with appropriate occupation, behavioural abnormalities might be largely or entirely avoided together with the associated functional disruptions that would otherwise require remediation. If so, what may remain would be a range of conditions whose nature may be much clearer once the effects of lack of physiological and psychological 'exercise' had receded. Such an approach also holds the promise of providing fresh insights into the significance of positive experiences to animals.

Standardized Behavioural Testing in Non-Verbal Humans and Other Animals

6.1 Animal Welfare Relates to Subjective Experiences and Underlying Capacities

As already enumerated (Chapters 1 and 5), an animal's welfare is its overall state, whether that is good, neutral or bad. In recent years, this judgement has come to be dominated or defined by an attempt to appreciate the animal's own experiences. Intense negative experiences, for example pain and fear, represent some of the least ambiguous states of compromised welfare, and those with which we have the highest degree of empathy and which are likely to be linked to severe challenges to fitness (Fraser and Duncan, 1998). Reducing the negative experiences of the worst-affected members of a group (Ryder, 1998) or reducing the net suffering of the group as a whole (Singer, 1990) are both legitimate major concerns of animal welfare.

Animal welfare policy and practice are currently strongly based upon 'science', and in many cases science is represented by some kind of standardized test of subjective states. However, it is important to question the received and accepted meanings of these tests of fear, pain, stress and other such states. Many of these tests are, objectively speaking, very simple, and it is well within the capacity of most observers to decide for themselves, independently, both objectively and intuitively, how they should be interpreted. It is also often helpful to consider how and why the test was originally invented, how well it has subsequently been validated and whether it has drifted without appropriate modification from its original purpose and application.

6.1.1 Standardized tests are intuitive attempts to capture a subjective state in a single, empirical index

The genesis of any particular objective/empirical test intended to capture an animal's subjective state tends to be an intuitive leap made by a person with a specific problem at hand. A person familiar with the species and the goal of the test will generally focus on something that 'makes sense' on the basis of ethological face value. Thus, rats are tested in a large open 'field' which might elicit variable amounts of anti-predator freezing depending on how much the animal's genetics and prior experience have inclined it to react fearfully to this challenge (Hall, 1934). The subjective/intuitive basis of test design is not a flaw so long as the test itself is objective/empirical and is treated as an expert hypothesis which every data set will support, or fail to support. The credibility and usefulness of each test depend on it being constantly assessed for its limits in terms of context and predictive value.

For example, Welp *et al.* (2004) did not use an open field to assess fear in cows as there is no ethological basis for suggesting that they become motionless to avoid predation. Instead, they suggested that when cows are more fearful they will be more vigilant at the expense of feeding from an attractive food source. The cows immediately demonstrated this variable's appropriate responsiveness to predator-like individuals such as dogs, and to unfamiliar or rough human handlers (compared with controls). However, as responses to a novel place were less clear the test's use to measure novel-place fearfulness is not yet supported. Accordingly, this vigilance test looks promising in having face validity, supportive data and current boundaries for appropriate use, for example quantifying variables reflecting fear of dogs and humans. From here it might be assessed for insensitivity to factors that should

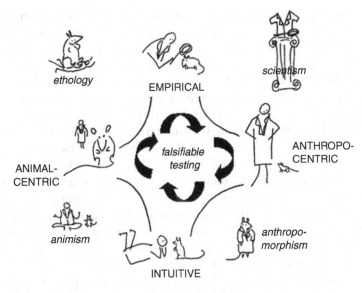

Figure 6.1 Schema of balanced conceptual positions for behavioural testing.

not affect fear, and perhaps also for its predictive value, for instance for identifying animals that will be more stressed during intensive handling procedures such as hoof-trimming.

Each behavioural test should maintain a balanced conceptual position; where falsifiable, empirical testing plays a central role (Figure 6.1).

- It should be *animalcentric* to an extent that springs from an understanding of some functional response of the animal to specific stimuli and a plausibly associated subjective state.
- It should be *anthropocentric* in that this behaviour is assessed with a certain human goal in mind.
- It should be *intuitive* in that the emotional state captured and the motivation of the animal must be understood through a degree of empathy.
- And it should be *empirical* in that the data collected are objective and either support or do not support the presumed nature of the test.

For effective testing in any arena of animal use, all four of these perspectives must be taken into consideration in a balanced way. Errors are most likely to occur when there is an over-reliance on one or two aspects combined with a failure to subject any approach to falsifiable testing. The most widely discussed error in test construction and use is *anthropomorphism*. For example, assuming an animal will benefit from conditions that humans enjoy, leading to conditions that do not meet species-specific needs, such as providing a very clean open cage to mice, which will tend to prefer having a familiar-smelling place in which to hide.

Anthropomorphism is not a failure *because* it is intuitive and empathetic; rather, it is a failure *of* that faculty in assuming animals will like what people would like, an assumption that is sometimes true and sometimes not. This intuition can be corrected by balancing it with *animalcentric* intuitions from animal-familiar experts, and through collection of data designed to allow the animal to express its own perspective, such as through preference testing or a stress response.

A good test-development system will lead to the correction of false intuitions not only about the nature of animal emotional responses (Are they like ours or different?), but also about the nature of the scientific test (Does it measure what we think it does, or not?). The data collected should be such that the measured variables are clearly relevant to the subjective state, for example variables that should cause more fear in the rat should cause more freezing in the open field. However, in some cases allegiance of testers to a test prevents potentially falsifying data from being collected or confronted. Thus, anomalies are explained away as being due to poor technique and tests become encumbered with irrelevant requirements in order to get the 'right' results.

This is not to say that unbalanced combinations are wrong in general, just that they are outside the realm of standardized testing for the purposes of refinement. 'Unbalanced' approaches may meet other goals – for example, research about the animal for its own sake (ethological/conservation-oritented research) – or may relate to animistic religion-based feelings about animals that are spiritual (subjectively 'true' perceptions) rather than to hypothetical constructs subject to consensus-based validation.

6.1.2 Standard tests for general traits such as temperment or emotionality have great limitations

It is enough of a challenge to try to assess the presence or degree of an extant emotional state, yet a great deal more is often required. When environments cannot be brought fully under control attention fastens more on producing animals which, through their genetics and early experience, are equipped to cope with the unavoidable or necessary challenges of their environment. Such animals are intelligent and proactive enough to acquire the resources that they need, yet placid enough to avoid unnecessary anxiety and not represent a danger to others. These are presumed to be general, long-term or even lifelong traits that it would be useful to quantify for appropriate placement of individuals and breeding of lines. Thus, standardized testing attempts to capture not only what an animal feels in a given moment, but what it possesses in terms of temperament or personality.

One of the difficulties in this area is the tendency to use existing tests, rather than develop new approaches from scratch through a fresh intuition about the animal/purpose being studied. Thus, researchers using or reviewing research based on human personality tests tend to find that animals have personalities like humans, but are missing or deficient in certain areas (Gosling and John, 1999). This reinforces a fallacy, common in psychology, that animals have 'all the processes found in man ... in simpler forms' as opposed to possessing some processes common to various other species and some very complex ones entirely of their own (Mehlmen, 1967, p. 70).

Meanwhile, researchers adapting tests developed with rodents tend to find that personality is based primarily on a dimension of 'emotionality', which is now often called 'fearfulness'. Note, however, that the primary trait with rats is arguably exploration, with fear coming in at second place (Markel, 1999). The meaning of tests 'of' emotionality tends to vary between different strains and species of rodent, for example with fear that sometimes causes freezing and sometimes flight, and defaecation that sometimes relates to fear and sometimes to territory marking. Denenberg (1969) used the open-field test with an awareness that its meaning must be ascertained and the limits of that meaning understood:

'... the operational definition of an emotional animal is one that has a low activity score and a high defecation score.... My statements are reasonable, they have ethological validity – and they are, of course, completely circular. We can state, if we wish, that emotionality is that which the open-field measures and feel safe, secure and smug behind such a statement. If we do this, however, we are avoiding one quite unpleasant aspect of reality: how do we demonstrate the validity of the statement that the open field test measures the construct of emotionality?'

And upon ascertaining that validity to his own satisfaction he still warns:

'... all of this validation was obtained within the context of early experience research.... However, this does not mean the same conceptual meanings may be attributed ... in other research contexts.'

Let alone, one must add, to other species.

With the passage of time this reliance on explicit validation within prescribed boundaries seems to have largely faded from use. And the validation studies that do exist have mixed success such that the existence of an underlying fearfulness trait even in rats and mice cannot be considered proven, let alone in other species such as dogs where it is the most frequently examined temperament dimension by virtue of the adoption of rodent-based methodologies (Jones and Gosling, 2005). The notion of emotionality as an animal personality trait (see Hall, 1934; Denenberg, 1964) has always suffered from 'a gulf between theory and empirical data' (Archer, 1973), a gulf that has continued to expand as the notion has been more widely applied and less frequently subject to direct scrutiny. It seems that as the invention of a test falls from living memory it is increasingly assumed by those in need of behavioural tools that the test is broadly and robustly valid when, historically speaking, this was never established.

And just to confuse matters further, there is a separate and more modern theory of the fundamental nature of rodent personality that asserts that there are two distinct personality 'types': proactive and reactive. This development seems to suggest that even rodent-based tests reflect more *our perspective* on rodent personality than the tests' reality for the rodent. Consider that the usual response to humans by ungentled rats is anti-predatory, and that rats carried to the open field in their cages rather than by hand, or previously gentled rats, often display little or no fear in the open field (e.g. Spence and Maher, 1962). Thus, 'emotionality' may have less to do with how rodents see the world in general, and more about how they see us in particular, and not very positively at that. The general scientific response to this finding was to always perform the open field first in a series of tests, rather than in a randomized counterbalanced order, and to generally avoid handling outside of test procedures; that is, to add requirements that should be irrelevant to long-term 'personality' traits in order to get the 'right' test results.

Based on the newer proposition of personality types, tests were developed for agricultural animals such as chickens and pigs. An early description of the so-called pig back test, which quantifies struggling when piglets are held lying on their backs, led to an assertion that pigs are, generally and probably according to a binomial distribution, identifiable as active or passive cope-ers, and that these traits could be reliably measured early in life. This idea persists despite many later studies questioning its validity with the outcomes of the back test being only sporadically related to those of other tests and not very stable over time. There are certainly traits other than coping style that may be more important in understanding livestock temperament on its own terms, for example aggressiveness (Ruis *et al.*, 2000).

In turn, it must be noted that rodent emotionality is presumed to be a valid model for human anxiety, to the extent that anxiolytic medication may be tested using rodents. Yet this generalization is also questionable (Calatayud *et al.*, 2004). Although this rodent model seems to adequately represent normal human anxiety, it does not adequately represent the anxiety disorders most pharmaceuticals are intended to treat (Prut and Belzung, 2003).

In each case, there is a clear tendency to suggest that the subject's nature is what the researcher expected it to be, or what is traditionally measured. This is by no means new or surprising as those who cannot speak for themselves have always tended to have their behaviour interpreted to the benefit of those who can; for example, 'Kenneth Krechevsky's (1932) rats even back in the thirties had hypotheses, and Snygg's (1936) rats were apparently seen as phenomenologists, but these rats were clearly unrelated to Hull's "behavioristic" rats' (Mehlman, 1967).

6.2 Origins in Human Verbal Testing

6.2.1 Verbal human self-report is considered the most reliable way to detect negative states and impaired coping abilities

The first intuitive test of well-being in humans is to simply ask how someone is. However, it is important to understand that verbal behaviour, although able to represent uniquely complex information, is no more reliable than other responses in terms of accuracy. In fact, a wide variety of studies have determined that verbal reports that a human gives of their own behaviour have only a weak relationship to the actual, independently observed performance of this behaviour. Verbal identification (eye-witness reports) are equally unreliable. This is due occasionally to deliberate deceit, particularly when the person has a clear motivation to lie. But more often it is due to the fact that the verbal report relates not to the present situation but to memory of past events or intentions for future behaviours, neither of which are as reliable as is commonly assumed.

However, where a current state is being reported, and causes of deceit are minimized, self-report is a convenient way to access a human's subjective world. This realization, over time, led to the formulation of standardized questions for health-care professions. And when the more chronic and general states are of concern, for example general anxiety rather than current fear, self-report tends to be aggregated into a battery of tests using verbal questions and often verbal or written responses.

The flagship of standardized testing must be the questionnaire. This initial bias towards question and answer represented an immediate challenge to the validity of such testing, as a reliance on spoken or written language is not merely anthropocentric but privileges all those who grasp the language employed as fully and in the same way as those who create and deliver the test. For example, the dramatic increase in average IQ that has been observed across the last several decades may be related to an increased tendency for modern people to use abstract rather than concrete concepts, so the general public is now more familiar with the 'scientifically correct' answer to questions open to multiple interpretations (Gladwell, 2007). Even non-verbal test components rely heavily on the comprehension of spoken instructions about how these features should be manipulated or interpreted.

Thus, test scores tend to implicitly support the intuitive understanding of those who created the test, such that their own verbal in-group is both superior (i.e. more intelligent) and more sensitive (i.e. more apt to suffer from poor treatment). By limiting data to language channels potentially contradictory information of other types is excluded or 'trumped'. The result can be seen in the role of professionals in contributing to stereotyped beliefs relating to race, class, nationality, age and gender (see Guthrie, 1998).

6.2.2 It is very widely believed that without fully realized language individuals are by definition less capable of suffering or possess impaired intellect

There are two main ways in which humans are characterized. One is what we consider central to our natures (separating us from machines), and the other is what can be used to distinguish us from the organisms most similar to us (animals; Haslam, 2006). Language seems to come up in the latter case because complex, syntactical language is difficult to perceive in animals. Although various animals such as birds and apes have mastered, to some extent, abstract words and syntax (Gentner *et al.*, 2006), it has never risen, even in the case of primates, to the level of what could truly be considered inter-species *'conversation'* (Dekkers, 2000). A restrictive definition of language remains one of the strongest candidates for defining humans as different from other animals (Premack, 2004).

Nevertheless, most people consider animals to possess minds, and based on this 94% of college students reported talking to companion animals 'in the manner of talking to a person' (Rasmussen and Rajecki, 1995). There seems to be an intuitive belief that meaningful communication between species is possible, albeit unproductive in view of the insistence that it should take the form of spoken human language. Whereas core theory in animal welfare science explicitly emphasizes suffering over intelligence (Dawkins, 1998), many scientists are apparently willing to disregard the interests of animals that are not capable, somehow, of comprehending the intent of spoken language. For example: 'The problem is, there is a range of sentience.... I can talk ugly to my dog, and he'll sulk away. If I talk ugly to a chicken, he'll just look at me. The bottom line is that legal rights should only be afforded to species that can comprehend that concept' (Irvin, 2007).

Failures of communication are typically ascribed by the human listener *to* the animal speaker, rather than as shared inadequacies. For example, 'It is even more difficult to identify and measure pain in animals, as their communication capacities are much less' (Anonymous, 2004). From there it is a short step to the assertion that self-awareness will not develop without language, and fundamental experiences such as pain are not experienced as intensely or at all by individuals that are not self-aware. This belief is especially prevalent when it is convenient or beneficial to the one who holds it. Although in our general day-to-day interactions, belief in animals having minds leads to attempts to communicate with them, equally *within science* failed attempts to communicate conversationally have led to arguments against animals being completely sentient.

Piglets are an example of the crucial difference between being non-verbal (unable to communicate) and non-lingual (unable to converse in human fashion). They produce vocalizations including a 'scream' that is more frequent and of different pitch when being castrated rather than when they are simply held; also there are associated escape attempts and signs of physiological stress (e.g. Taylor and Weary, 2000; Marx *et al.*, 2003). As such, these utterances must be considered to be 'words' that communicate a meaning ('that hurts') with a great degree of clarity for those attending to the scream, so piglets are indeed verbal. They simply do not use words spoken in a human language, although their 'words' are arguably part of a cross-species *lingua franca* of hostile, friendly and fearful sounds that, in such contexts, we have apparently actively learned to ignore or misinterpret (Morton, 1977). These are exactly the kinds of 'honest' inter-species signals upon which tests should be based.

Human infants, on the other hand, may not always vocalize in response to pain, especially premature babies who may have impaired lung development.

However, they do make great use of the non-verbal equivalent of the pain scream, the grimace. For a long time premature infants were very closely monitored and manipulated under bright lights, and blood samples might be taken several times a day via a 'heel stick'. Two considerations led to the development of less stressful conditions in wards for pre-term babies. One was an appreciation of the 'ethology' of pre-term babies, which would normally be developing in the dark and insulated environment of the womb (see Chapter 10). The other was training staff in a renewed sensitivity to grimace and withdrawal responses. A regime of compulsory sampling effectively trained nurses to disregard and de-emphasize the meaning of these responses in order to carry out these tasks without experiencing much distress themselves. However, when they were empowered to heed the meaning of a grimace, rapid changes in procedure occurred, and sampling was performed only when necessary, incubators were blanket-draped to darken them and sounds, lights and disturbances were minimized.

Because of the perceived or implicit connection between the use of language and the ability to suffer, or to be considered at all, there are now entire areas of research devoted to contradicting the assumption that no language equals no welfare. These can be divided roughly into programmes attempting to teach a human language to an animal, such as sign language to chimpanzees and gorillas, and those trying to find other gestural equivalents of self-awareness, such as evidence that an animal can recognize itself in a mirror. However, in this case science may be trying to solve a problem caused only by its own culture. If conversational language is not deemed necessary for suffering it is far simpler to communicate using the signals the animals is already predisposed to emit. After all, if we really want to hear what the animal has to say the burden is placed upon us to comprehend the message already being sent, not on the animal to 'speak properly'.

Standardized testing depends upon eliciting and comprehending the animal's (and non-verbal human's) innate language, be it auditory, gestural, odour, electrical or some other form, and upon finding a way to render it into our own speech without losing too much in translation.

6.3 Appreciating the Suffering and Capacities of Humans with Impaired Self-Report

Impaired communication is often due to little more than limited opportunities to interact. Structures, by design or accident, tend to limit the time those who will cause pain, no matter how necessary, spend with those who will experience it, for example between surgeon and patient. In addition, the language used by doctors between themselves is very accurate for their purposes, but often lacks clarity for patients who may fail to understand even basic instructions. A recent study determined that lay understanding of medical terms is often weak, and lay listeners are often over-confident in rating their own comprehension (Chapman et al., 2003).

Difficulties become more pronounced with those humans who are actually incapable of comprehending or producing grammatical speech, for example infants or those suffering from dementia or schizophrenia (DeLisi, 2001). Repeated studies have shown that those unable to verbally request care such as pain relief are less likely to receive it. Likewise, those less able to verbally protest impositions are less likely to avoid them. In both cases, the non-verbal channels of communication may be fully employed, but without effect.

6.3.1 Proxies

There seems to be a need to assiduously ensure that caretakers of non-verbal humans are attending to other methods of communication. One of the simplest approaches to this has been the use of verbal proxies who essentially 'translate' the individual's need(s) into words. There seems to be little doubt that interested persons such as friends and parents can advocate for patients and so counter pressures that might otherwise deprive them of needed care. While it is doubtful that these proxies will always have a good appreciation of the individual's subjective state, they may certainly cause it to be under greater scrutiny. Proxies familiar with animals will tend to be their legal owners who may have a vested interest in exploiting them, whereas 'stranger' animal advocates may lack the ethological knowledge or personal relationship with the animal needed for accurate empathy. However, the mere presence of human proxies raises the question of what the animal actually is experiencing and so may lead to the detection of lapses in care.

6.3.2 Scales

In order to assess the accuracy of a proxy's reports, they need to be fixed on a numerical scale and compared with other measures to which they should relate. It must be noted that use of a scale formalizes the intensity of a state but does not make this estimate any more valid. There seems to be a tendency for procedures that produce numerical rather than qualitative outputs to be assumed to have greater scientific validity when, at best, they are more amenable to being tested for this quality. It must also be understood that empirical scales sacrifice semantic value in the process of being fixed, and there is a danger that the actual meaning of the scale may be assigned somewhat arbitrarily by the enumerator.

6.3.3 Behavioural tests

An advantage of behavioural tests is that the information collected comes directly from the individual under scrutiny. Often the tests simply quantify communication that has clear intuitive value. For example, individuals in pain may grimace and show other expressions. These data may then be compared with other measures such as physiological stress and self-administration of relieving agents, as well as to future outcomes.

When the trait being measured is more diffuse, like an aptitude for a task, a wider battery of measures is taken. In this case, the main challenge of the tests is not the authenticity of the responses, but their relevance.

6.4 Questioning the Tests; Breakdowns in Communication

A correctly formulated standardized behavioural test allows an animal to give an accurate and relevant answer to a human question, such as: are you afraid? However, testing can also provide a false certainty. This occurs when the results generated are interpreted with reference to the intent of the test not the actual status of the animal. However, by regarding the test as a proxy for our more familiar forms of spoken communication, we can work critically on its flaws as a form of two-way communication, provided also that we attend to all of the animal's responses and compare their meaning with the stimulus provided and all potential explanations.

When a rat is placed in the open field we ask the question: are you afraid? But if a handler remains in the test room the rat tends to stay in the area nearest to her/him, thereby reducing its activity levels. Thus, it answers 'yes' but to the question 'do you like/trust your handler?' Similarly, behaviours in the same environment might still have different causes with an increased activity in one strain of rat being frantic escape attempts, and in another confident exploration of a novel area. Behaviours do not have a fixed and unvarying meaning; they must always be read anew and interpreted in context, even under ostensibly standardized conditions. A failure to understand that our 'reading' of behaviour is often unreliable, and easily biased, readily leads to improper uses of behavioural tests. We have a great many ways of measuring what animals do, but seem to neglect the equally important and ongoing task of observing *how* – that is, in what manner – they do it, and *deciding* why we think they are doing it, rather than assuming that we already know, or that, somehow, the test knows.

6.4.1 Dead dogs tell no tales: temperament testing in animal shelters

Dogs are tested to select them for vocations such as police or guide dog work. Over time successive, purpose-bred generations have performed better at the tests, but not at the work. It is not possible to know how dogs that fail the tests would fare in the vocations, but these results do not give cause for confidence.

A more extreme potential example of failed dog-temperament testing can be found in the widespread use of 'temperament' tests in shelters. Dogs that respond by snarling or biting, for example to having food taken from them, may be placed with more experienced owners who are likely to able to correct this behaviour. However, given the high numbers of homeless adult dogs, and the potential legal liability of the shelters for injuries, many 'failing' dogs will be euthanized rather than re-homed. Thus, the validity of the test for predicting aggression in the future home is not subject to challenge, so the basis for selecting dogs to be euthanized may remain spurious. If faith in the test has developed, this represents an injustice to those animals that fail, an injustice of which the decision-maker will be unaware. It may also be emotionally less challenging to consider animals that are actually euthanized for reasons of space or cost as unsuitable as pets – that is, 'unadoptable' – especially if the choice to kill can be made to seem less arbitrary (not based on breed, colour or passage of time). In this way, *practical* and *emotional* goals are met but the *animal's* needs are not.

Failure to expose temperament tests to actual falsifiability assessment, especially for failing dogs, is rendered an even greater error when these tests proliferate and are offered as paid services by experts with a financial reason to avoid challenges to their product's validity. Parallels might be drawn to human tests, especially those employed to manage large groups of people. For example, originally IQ tests had the goal of directing extra education to under-performing children but instead, under commercial pressure, they quickly became a way to deny opportunities to those deemed unlikely to benefit from them, and to allow human resource departments to screen applicants and perpetuate their own professional role. They started as a test of the failures of the eduation system, and ended up as an indictment of the child's innate worth.

To counterbalance the convenience value of screening out aggressive dogs, shelters might consider publicly reporting failure rates and following up any cases where failing animals were re-homed for comparison with dogs that passed. The test should be scrutinized for correlation with irrelevant factors. For example, the pressure to euthanize at a shelter may effectively determine how well a dog needs to score to survive. It should never actually affect how well any given dog scores on the test or what proportion are deemed objectively to 'fail'; this should relate only to them being a danger to future owners, and this conclusion cannot be confidently drawn as it is not subject to test.

The value of a test is never greater than its outcome. Therefore, all tests should be trusted only to the extent that these outcomes are measured and conform to expectations. In the case of dog-aggression tests, evidence is weak for the success of test-passers and entirely absent for the failure of test-failers, and neglects the potential beneficial impact of appropriate behavioural management and modification. Also, a behaviour never presupposes its own cause or intractability. Snapping or growling by dogs may well be due to transient states such as new-place and isolation stress, excessive hunger or fear. Aggression caused more diffusely may respond to treatment, or the dog may be placed in an environment that lacks the required 'triggers' (Winograd, 2005). We must challenge the very idea that temperament testing tests temperament; in fact, it tests behaviour. The contribution of stable and unalterable personality traits will be variable, may be low, and certainly cannot be judged based on the test alone.

So what can shelter staff do? Clearly it is wise to undertake a degree of behaviour testing, but preferably over time and incorporating ongoing habituation and training and a range of experiences. However, in the absence of a validated temperament test, determining whether a dog is adoptable must remain a judgement, one that staff make based on their training and intuition, their relationship with the animal and their moral duty to the future owner and society. Dressing this decision up in the suits of science is a fiction, because the so-called science is unproven, produces fallacy not accuracy and entrenches beliefs that, for instance, one snap indicates a permanently aggressive personality because the very nature of the test implies this interpretation no matter what disclaimers may be attached. Where the science is unproven human judgement must trump unreliable numbers, explicitly and without exception, because such human judgement, even when unproven as a predictor, is innately more broadly based and a matter of personal responsibility, doubt and contemplation for the people who make it. Basing such judgement on direct observation and a relationship with an animal is innately more thoughtful, whereas standardized behavioural tests seem too often to become a substitute for thought and the employment of highly competent and empowered staff.

Finally, consider honestly, is it not so that in most cases the reason the dogs are being killed is our creation of a system of over-supply and lack of resources, not the unworthiness of the dogs? In this case, the old system of euthanizing by age, appearance and length of stay may actually be the correct one, and temperament testing may be a step backwards towards suggesting somehow that the basic problem with re-homing stray dogs rests primarily with the dogs themselves not our management of them. If less 'appealing' or over-supplied types and colours of dogs and those that are not attracting interest are removed, the remaining pool of puppies, mainly small and attractive dogs, may generate more adoptions, maximizing the number saved. Consideration of behavioural problems, not limited to aggression, could be more appropriately directed at minimizing 'returns' or other relinquishment and optimizing the number of successful adoptions in the long term.

6.5 Conclusions: Trust the Animal not the Test

We have developed many tests that have, under some conditions, aided us in understanding animals' subjective states. However, the meaning of the test on *every single* new occasion remains at the level of an hypothesis, so that each test should always be used in a manner where this meaning is falsifiable or at least open to question and alternative explanations. The nature of the test hypothesis and its appropriateness must be explicit, and must be subject to critical scrutiny.

A test maze may under some circumstances measure a quality in rats that could be called intelligence. However, more fearful rats perform more poorly; those given electric shocks or starved to hurry them do better. Likewise, although, all other things being equal, a more fearful rat will be less active in an open field and tend to stay close to the wall, an open field is not a test of fear. Activity levels may be increased without any likely effect on fearfulness by feeding the animal more or removing its vibrissae (something that might happen unintentionally, such as through barbering) (Prut and Belzung, 2003). Likewise, a blind chicken pecks other hens less often but cannot meaningfully be said to be less aggressive as a temperament trait, although dim contact lenses that injure the eyes of hens have indeed been sold based on the argument that less pecking can only mean less aggression and better welfare (Gvaryahu and Snapir, 1997). We should attribute meaning to animals' behaviours as we observe them and immediately afterwards, taking into account all we observe and based on a minimum effective understanding of the species and the individual, not at the point of test selection. Unless the experiment is designed to allow falsifiability of the preferred meaning, the interpretation is a leap of faith not an act of science.

It is hoped that the standardized nature of the test will allow us to predetermine the nature of the variable being measured. However, not only does this not cover conditions where independent or intervening variables are deliberately changed, as exact replication is of little value, but also ones where they differ unintentionally. Our ability to achieve actual standardization appears to be very low even with well-known tests. For instance, with almost every reported use the open field varies its size, shape, lighting and duration, and these are only the reported variables. Even when every effort is made to make the apparatus, animals and procedure uniform, different laboratories fail to replicate even the direction of effect (Crabbe *et al.*, 1999). The widespread impression that standardized tests are valid and robust may be largely an illusion, but without frequent attempts to falsify the dominant interpretation of each test it is difficult to be sure.

When the exact nature of the animal's response is known and robustly valid, including a firm knowledge of valid environmental causes, variation of all other features of the environment should be able to occur freely. For example, Grandin (1998) suggested that if a slaughterhouse floor was too slippery animals would fall, and when the situation was too frightening they would vocalize. These relationships may be employed with tolerable success in any slaughterhouse regardless of construction. Both of these measures are in fact standardized behavioural tests which are arguably more reliable than many used under controlled laboratory conditions. The degree of standardization of a test is far less important than its focus. Thus, any test that requires standardization of variables *that should not be relevant* is almost certainly not valid even when the results perfectly match our expectations.

In short, although we attempt to use standardized behavioural tests as a method of communication to replace spoken language, our success to date is not encouraging. This is not only because our questions are poorly formed, but because we are failing to attend to the answers and continue the dialogue in both directions. The first step in the development of any test should be to act like a traveller in a foreign land, ready to learn the language and customs of its people, not a conqueror arriving to impose his own way of life.

In both human and non-human animal cases, special care must be taken not to lose communication with, and thereby care poorly for, groups where optimal care is inconvenient for us and they are powerless to demand it. They include infants, 'workers', the mentally ill, homeless populations and any vulnerable individual without an expert advocate of some kind who acts primarily as their proxy. They clearly also include the animals we use for our human purposes and often to their detriment.

Research encompassing non-verbal individuals, both humans and other animals, has led to the realization that standardized tests are often flawed and require constant vigilance to attain and maintain any validity. The use of formal, standard and objective methods does not, in itself, assure validity. It is clear, therefore, that false confidence in the validity of a test with objective, empirical, standardized properties (scientism) should be seen as just as dangerous as false confidence in empathy (anthropomorphism), if not more so.

Tests should be standardized, but equally they should constantly change to adapt to every minute variation in context to keep the message 'in focus'. Moreover, we need to recognize that the ultimate delivery of appropriate care inevitably depends upon both the researcher/caretaker heeding, compassionately, the responses of their charges and their attempt to use science to better understand them in their own terms.

Part 4

Human Inputs and Animal Welfare

Human–Animal Interactions and Animal Welfare

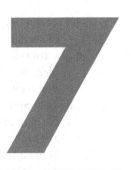

7.1 Introduction

7.1.1 Human–animal interactions reflect human needs and human attitudes towards animals and also whether animals meet those needs and affect those attitudes

Humans are an important part of the environment of domesticated animals in terms of both the control they exert over the environment and their physical presence in it. Human behaviour towards animals is affected by human attitudes towards their own physical, economic, social, religious and other needs. Domestication itself is a generic form of human needs-based behaviour. Over millennia, it has resulted in the production, from original species, of many breeds of animal whose characteristics have been designed to meet particular human needs. Animal characteristics in their turn influence human attitudes, and these have impact on how animals are managed. For instance, cattle in Europe are farmed as production animals to provide milk and meat and are regarded as economic entities. In contrast, cattle have a much wider role in some African societies, such as the Nuer, where they are fundamental to physical survival, but they are also the basis of social life and the focus of poetry and song (Willis, 1974). Thus, although cattle produce milk and meat for both communities the attitudes towards them are quite different depending on the physical and socio-cultural environment.

Socio-cultural and anthropological studies of human–animal relationships recognize that animals may be a focus of conflict, being variously regarded as commodities, family members, food, prey, entertainment and a representative of nature (Mullins, 1999). These conflicts are predictable given the diversity of contexts in which people interact with individual species. For instance, the dog may be a family member, the focus of nurturing human behaviour, a major source of emotional support or a co-worker (e.g. service dogs) for some people, yet it may also be a source of food, motive power or entertainment, or a research tool, a nuisance or a pest for others (Stafford, 2006). The outcomes of socio-cultural research, in being generally anthropocentric, may do little for our understanding of animal welfare beyond helping us to understand different human perspectives. Indeed, a major dichotomy in human attitudes towards animals has emerged: one element is centred on the notion that animal behaviour is predominantly reactive, a response to the environment, and the other on the idea that it is largely self-generated and active. The former implies mainly a mechanical, less emotionally sensitive response, while the latter suggests a subjective more sensitive life experience, with each having different implications for what treatment is considered to be reasonable for animals.

American attitudes towards animals have been characterized and evaluated by Kellert (1988). Neutralistic (avoid animals) and humanistic (appreciate pets) attitudes, which are quite different and almost opposite, were equally common, followed by utilitarian and moralistic attitudes, which again are almost opposite and equally common (Table 7.1). Such commonly held and differing attitudes may help to explain the often diametrically opposed perspectives reflected in the multiplicity of interactions observable between humans and animals.

In this chapter, our understanding of domestication, which is the basis of human interactions with all domestic animals, will be discussed in the context of animal welfare. This will be followed by discussion of the welfare implications of the interaction between humans and farm livestock, companion animals and animals used in sport and entertainment.

Table 7.1 The attitudes of Americans towards animals (Kellert, 1988). Reproduced with permission from Stephen R. Kellert.

Attitude	Percentage of population	Common expression
Humanistic	35	Strong affection for individual animals; anthropomorphic
Neutralistic	35	Disinterested in animals and avoids them
Utilitarian	20	Interest in practical value of animals
Moralistic	20	Concern for right and wrong treatment of animals
Aesthetic	15	Interest in attractiveness and symbolic appeal of animals
Naturalistic	10	Interest and affection for animals and outdoors
Ecologistic	7	Concern for environment and animal habitats
Dominionistic	3	Interest in control of animals
Negativistic	2	Dislike of animals
Scientific	1	Interest in form and function of animals

7.2 Domestication

7.2.1 Domestication may be understood using various paradigms that incorporate presumed human–animal interactions in antiquity

A wide range of scientists and others, including anthropologists, economists and social scientists, have studied the process of domestication (Price, 2002). Those scholars have variously considered domestication to be a predominantly human-initiated activity carried out for non-materialistic ritual reasons where particular animals, for instance, were taken to embody different forms of divine, spiritual or natural power, or for economic self-sustaining purposes where animals were seen primarily as a source of food, clothing, draught power, protection and so on. Conversely, more recently domestication has been evaluated as an animal-initiated, ecologically constrained activity. According to this paradigm, domestication of the wolf, the first animal to be domesticated, was probably initiated by young wolves which, after being driven from their natal territory, came to live near humans where they gradually became part of the fabric of camp life. The selection of wolves capable of living and reproducing close to human encampments was probably influenced by the natural characteristics of individual animals and by the response of humans to them. Thus, two forms of selection were probably in play: natural selection towards those wolves that were more at ease living near encampments, and artificial selection by humans who chose those wolves that would be allowed to live within their camp and rejected those that would not. Such selection by humans may not have been driven by economic factors but by recognition that wolf behaviour towards visitors was useful.

The wolf became the dog 10 millennia before the next species, sheep and goats, were domesticated. Thus, there is little need to posit that the process was similar for all species. Moreover, the environmental, social and economic factors that may have influenced the domestication of sheep and goats may have differed from those that led to the subsequent domestication of cattle and other livestock. Much more recent human-initiated domestication activities appear to have been driven by specific requirements such as a need for laboratory rats or by a desire for red deer to replace sheep on some hill farms in New Zealand (Figure 7.1).

7.2.2 Understanding the process of domestication may lead to breeding strategies that will improve animal welfare during future attempts at domestication

Understanding the mechanisms of domestication may, in future, enable additional species to be domesticated in controlled ways that allow their efficient modification, as desired, but with an emphasis on minimizing negative welfare consequences.

The behavioural and physical changes brought about by domestication have been identified (Price, 2002). As already noted, the fundamental behavioural change is an ability to live healthy lives and reproduce in proximity to human beings. Physical

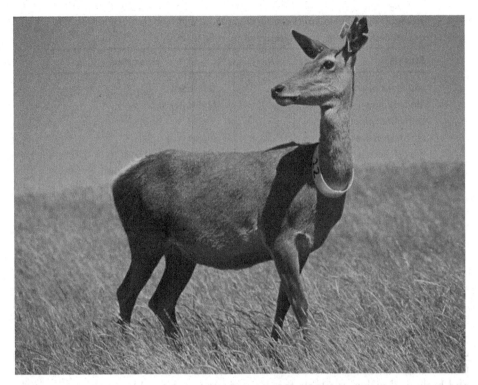

Figure 7.1 Red deer hind on a New Zealand farm (©2009, M.W. Fisher, reproduced with permission).

changes include an initial reduction in size, some changes to skull morphology and perhaps coat colour. Also, domestic animals retain some of the social characteristics of juvenile members of the progenitor species, such as attention-seeking and playful behaviour in dogs. The modification of species post-domestication to fulfil specific roles and suit particular environments by selective breeding has further changed domesticated animals. Extreme examples of physical changes with negative welfare consequences are seen in the modern English bulldog (McGreevy and Nicholas, 1999; Chapter 4), Belgian Blue cattle and some mice produced with specific genetic aberrations.

Research showing that domestication can have positive welfare outcomes has been conducted by biological scientists, such as Belyaev in the former Soviet Union who worked with initially wild foxes (Trut, 1999). By selecting annually 4–5% of males and 20% of females based on their behaviour towards humans, and breeding from them, Belyaev found, over a 40-year period, that he could produce a population of foxes in which 70–80% were friendly towards humans. This illustrates that with intensive selection for ease and confidence around humans it is possible to 'domesticate' some species reasonably quickly. It also suggests that such selection may be used in future to reduce the stress of human contact and any associated animal-welfare compromise in additional species we may want near us.

Table 7.2 Behavioural characteristics of mammals which make them suited or unsuited to domestication (adapted from Price, 2002).

Suited	Unsuited
Large social units	Territorial
Male affiliated with social group	Males live separately
Dominance hierarchy	
Not aggressive	Aggressive
Promiscuous	Pair-bonding
Young mature at birth	Young immature at birth
Readily habituated to humans	Poorly habituated to humans
Short flight distance from humans	Long flight distance from humans
Small home range	Large home range
Omnivorous or generalist feeder	Specialized diet
Wide environmental tolerance	Narrow environmental tolerance
Not shelter-seeking	Shelter-seeking
Limited agility	Highly agile

Of all the mammalian and avian species available, few have been domesti-cated. This was possibly due to many species not being amenable to domestication (Table 7.2), but it may also reflect the limited number of suitable social, economic and biological niches available for domesticated animals. Moreover, once a niche had been filled there may have been little human motivation to domesticate another species for the same niche. For instance, why in antiquity would people consider domesticating other small ruminants once domesticated sheep and goats had filled particular niches? In the modern era in New Zealand, farming of red deer, which is a much larger ruminant than sheep and goats, has been undertaken for economic purposes. The species is being changed behaviourally, as aggressive behaviour is being selected against, but although promising progress has been made it is not yet clear how successful this will be.

The progenitor species of many domesticated animals have become extinct, but closely related species still exist. Our knowledge of the behaviour of these species improves our understanding of the behavioural requirements of their domesticated relatives. As an example, once it was confirmed that the wolf was the progenitor of the domestic dog, knowledge of the wolf helped us to understand dog behaviour by helping to dispel spurious connections being made between dogs and other canids such as jackals and foxes. Studying the ecol-ogy and behaviour of existing progenitor species, or close relatives, contributes to our understanding of how the domesticated species should be managed to maximize their welfare.

It is often stated, and probably true, that there are more tigers held as pets than live in the wild (Figure 7.2). This observation and the worldwide concern for the

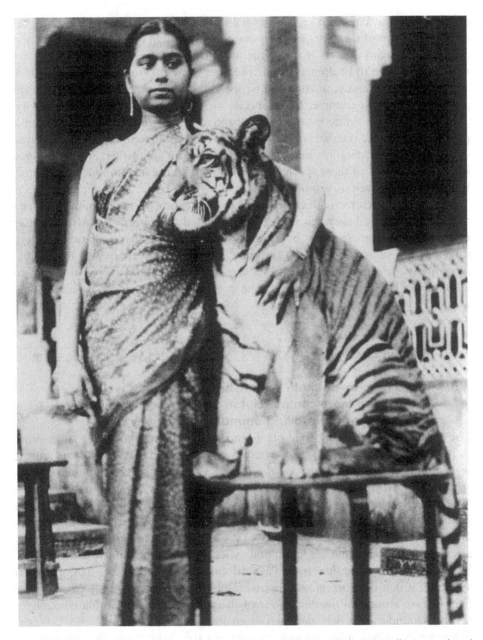

Figure 7.2 Teenage girl with her pet Bengal tiger, c. 1935 (©2009, D.J. Mellor, reproduced with permission).

preservation of endangered species has led to the development of programmes for the management of such species in captive colonies and in the wild. The wilderness available for many species is under threat, and the preservation of some species may require them to be domesticated. The tiger is an obvious case, in that with so many tigers in captivity, in zoos and parks, and owned as pets, there is room for a domestication programme. Many species are likely to survive only in captivity, and it seems appropriate to move from captive management to domestication if possible. As the mammalian species which have been domesticated have survived successfully, domestication may be an effective tool for preserving endangered species. However, for those species not amenable to domestication the process may be unsuitable on welfare grounds.

Our current scientific understanding of domestication allows unsuitable species to be identified, and domestication of those suited to the process. Also, we may now accelerate domestication by artificial insemination, super-ovulation, embryo transfer from suitable animals to surrogate mothers and perhaps also by cloning. Appropriate selection to modify responses to captivity and close proximity to humans would be expected to reduce the stress experienced by many captive wild species.

7.3 Farmed Livestock

7.3.1 Close human–animal relationships that extend well beyond the mere commercial in pastoral societies may reveal ways of improving animal welfare

The domestication of major food plants and the development of arable agriculture to provide food from fertile land occurred before sheep, goats, cattle and camels were domesticated (see Zeder *et al.*, 2006). The availability of these livestock species allowed humans to utilize pastureland that was less suitable for crops. Where land was more fertile initially, farmers probably tilled it for crops and also held livestock, but over time some farmers presumably favoured livestock farming and moved away to drier pastureland that was more suited to grazing. Additionally, as cropping land became overused, and yields declined, the land would still have been useful for grazing livestock. Pastoralists generally utilize one major animal species and one or more minor species. Thus, pastoralists in East Africa whose lives revolve around cattle may also own sheep, and people in Arabia whose lives revolve around camels may also own sheep and goats.

The study of pastoralist societies is usually carried out from an anthropological or ecological perspective. Willis (1974) delightfully described an exceptionally close relationship between people and their cattle. The Nuer people of southern Sudan depend on cattle for food and as a source of wealth to acquire brides, settle disputes and propitiate the spirits. But cattle also provide them with a poetic vocabulary and provide a focus for poetry and song (Willis, 1974). This understanding of the close interdependence between humans and cattle provides the basis for research into the manner in which humans and cattle have evolved to live symbiotically. It provides a basis for understanding the positive elements of animal welfare management when livestock, in this case cattle, are owned for more than merely commercial purposes.

Focusing on the *closeness* of interactions which may develop between people and livestock species such as cattle, but also horses, camels and pigs, may help us to clarify what is pleasurable for animals. The enjoyment which cattle experience when being fed particularly nutritious feedstuffs by their owner, and being sung to by them, could be an extreme variety of positive welfare (depending on the voice of the owner!) which merits further investigation by biologists.

7.3.2 Contemporary human interactions with farm livestock exhibit variable closeness with impacts on animals that are not wholly bad

The dependence of pastoralists on their grazing animals is profound, but dependence is also seen in subsistence farmers who need their traction animals such as oxen for cultivation and survival (Stafford, 1989). In modern large-scale commercial farming, however, frequent interactions between farmers and individual animals are not possible. Accordingly, animal relationships with humans currently range from the closeness of a man and his working oxen to the distance between a man and a cow defined as an economic unit, for instance, on a large ranch of thousands of cattle, where the essential focus is efficient food production. Farmers who have livestock or poultry may have to distance themselves from their animals in order to make the normal management of them easier. This is easier for farmers with large numbers of animals or birds but even farmers with few animals may try not to become too familiar with them to ease the negative experience of selling them for slaughter (Serpell, 1999). This focus may be set to change, however, as the cost of food becomes less important in many of the wealthy countries of the world and as management practices are increasingly engaging public interest. In addition, the role of farmers is changing from that of being only a food producer to that of food producer plus environmental guardian. A change in the public perception of farmers is likely as the latter become managers of eco-units with more objectives than food production alone (Nielsen, 1992).

It is not clear what role humans play in the interaction with farm animals from the animal's perspective. Humans may be perceived as a conspecific, existing within the animal's hierarchy as a boss animal, a friend animal or a substitute for offspring or mother. A second possibility is that humans may be perceived as a predator species controlling movement and behaviour, although this seems most unlikely in relationships such as those between a cow and her milker, or a calf and the person who feeds it. A third possibility related to benign interactions is that humans are perceived to be non-conspecifics and not predators; that is, they are perceived as different and non-threatening. Humans certainly control where animals can go and what they can do, but they may also play a role in giving the farm animal confidence and help it be content in its environment.

7.3.3 Understanding the basic fearfulness of farm animals and modifying human behaviour accordingly can enhance animal welfare and productivity

Although the process of domestication reduces the responsiveness of animals to humans, humans nevertheless remain a major source of fear and distress for some farm animals and poultry. The study of this aspect of the human–animal relationship has gone through a number of phases. Initially, Seabrook (1972) investigated the impacts of the psychological profiles or personalities of stockmen on animal productivity in the UK. Later, Hemsworth and Coleman (1998) investigated relationships between animal and human behaviour, and the impact of human attitudes and behaviour on animal productivity.

Seabrook (1972) found a relationship between the personality of the cowman and the mean herd milk yield. He observed that the cowmen he categorized as confident introverts were associated with higher yields. These individuals were identified as difficult to get on with and grumpy to co-workers, but their calm even-tempered and controlled nature around the animals may have had a positive impact on behaviour and productivity of dairy cows. Cowmen with extroverted personalities – active, excitable, lively, responsive and impulsive – were associated with lower milk yields. Thus, the behaviour of cowmen may not only affect the behaviour of the cows, but as indicated by the effects on milk yield it presumably also affects the animal's physiological state.

The behavioural and physiological responses of farm animals to human presence engaged the interest of animal scientists. Hemsworth and Barnett (1987) reported that on different farms pigs approached a human observer at varying time intervals after the observer initially entered the pigpen. They theorized that this variation in time to interact with humans was due to the pigs being influenced by the behaviour of the people working with them. The pig-orientated behaviour of people was categorized by Hemsworth and Coleman (1998) as negative or pleasant. Negative behaviours included forceful slaps, hits, kicks and pushes while positive behaviours included pats, strokes and a hand gently resting on the animal's back. They found that the greater the proportion of negative behaviours relative to the total number of tactile interactions, the longer it took for pigs to interact with people. This was attributed to greater levels of fear experienced by the negatively handled pigs. Depending on how they were handled, pigs differed in their behaviour, some physiological parameters and their productivity (Table 7.3). Hemsworth and Coleman (1998) developed a model relating human attitudes and behaviour toward animals to the fear, productivity, stress and levels of welfare of the animals.

Clearly, human behaviour can be of great significance to pigs when there are relatively close physical interactions between people and pigs. The behaviour of people working in poultry facilities also influences the behaviour and productivity

Table 7.3 The effects of handling behaviour on the time to interact with an observer, growth rate, plasma stress hormone (cortisol) levels and other parameters in pigs in four trials (adapted from Hemsworth and Barnett, 1987).

Type of handling	Pleasant	Minimal	Aversive
Trial 1			
Time to interact (s)	119		157
Growth rate (weeks 11–22) (g/day)	709		669
Cortisol levels (ng/ml)	2.1		3.1
Trial 2			
Time to interact (s)	73	81	147
Growth rate (weeks 8–18) (g/day)	897	888	837
Trial 3			
Time to interact (s)	10	92	160
Growth rate (weeks 7–13) (g/day)	455	458	404
Cortisol levels (ng/ml)	1.6	1.7	2.5
Trial 4			
Time to interact (s)	48	96	120
Pregnancy rate in gilts[a] (%)	88	57	33
Cortisol levels (ng/ml)	1.7	1.8	2.4

[a]Gilt: a maiden pig of breeding age.

of caged layer hens and broiler chickens. For instance, engaging in slow deliberate movements reduced avoidance behaviour (an indicator of fear) by hens in cages, and increased egg production (Barnett *et al.*, 1994).

A relationship between human behaviour and fearfulness and milk production in dairy cows has also been demonstrated (Breuer *et al.*, 2000). Fear of humans may have accounted for 19% of the variation in milk yield between farms. On farms where milk yield was low cows were less likely to approach humans. The way in which cattle are handled as calves at first milking and thereafter affects their response to humans (Hemsworth and Coleman, 1998), and unpleasant interactions may result in fear, and this in turn appears to influence plasma stress hormone (cortisol) levels. It is speculated that nervous cows with elevated cortisol levels may be immune-compromised and more prone to infectious disease. Yard and parlour design also influences the time cows take to enter the dairy parlour and may influence the nervousness of the cows (Fox, 1994). Cow-friendly, well-designed parlours may reduce stress and thereby improve health and welfare.

Thus, fear in farm animals of humans can have a negative impact on their productivity, for example with pigs, poultry and dairy cows, and a higher ratio of pleasant-to-negative behaviour by humans will have a positive impact on production, especially where an animal's contact with humans is high. In some countries, however, sheep and beef cattle are managed extensively and have little close contact with humans except when yarded for generally unpleasant experiences, for example ear-tagging, tail docking, castration, dehorning, shearing, vaccination, drenching, weaning, pregnancy diagnosis and drafting. Although sheep and beef cattle may see humans on a daily basis at a distance, the limited close contact and generally higher levels of fear experienced by these animals towards humans may in fact lessen the impact that human behaviour has on their productivity. However, this speculation needs to be quantified. In contrast, in sheep at least during lambing, the impact of human presence on fear may increase abandonment and mortality of lambs and thereby decrease productivity (Fisher and Mellor, 2002).

The fear that farm animals develop towards individual humans is usually generalized to a fear of all humans. Animals that have extensive, close and positive interactions with an individual human may discriminate between that person and others. Animals may learn to discriminate between humans who interact with them in a positive or negative manner particularly if the physical characteristics of the humans are distinct.

Finally, identifying the aspects of human interactions with animals which affect health may be important in preventing disease and injury. For instance, lameness of dairy cows is one disease condition that is directly influenced by human behaviour (Clarkson and Ward, 1991). In New Zealand, the major factors influencing the incidence of lameness in 62 herds in the Taranaki region were maintenance of farm tracks and farmer patience in not rushing the cows when bringing them in for milking (Chesterton *et al.*, 1989).

7.4 Companion Animals

7.4.1 Humans keep companion animals for many different reasons, which are usually human-centred

The levels of closeness between humans and animals vary considerably but closeness is seen most obviously in the interaction between humans and their companion animals or pets. The study of this closeness has been limited generally to survey research, the major focus of which has been on the impact of pets, especially dogs, on the physical and mental health of humans (see Robinson, 1995). The use of pets to help children with autism and other problems has been well documented. Also, the impact of interactions with animals on the quality of life of people in hospices, hospitals, psychiatric hospitals and prisons has been studied. In general, animals can be used to improve the lives of socially isolated people, and people who choose to own pets usually benefit from interacting with them. In contrast, the death and illness of an animal, or its misbehaviour, may have negative effects on the owner or caretaker.

During the last two decades there has been enormous interest in understanding why people keep pet animals. Studies have generally been by questionnaire and

Table 7.4 Reasons for owning or not owning a pet in descending order of importance (adapted from Leslie *et al.*, 1994).

Owning a pet	Not owning a pet
Companionship	A problem when I go away
Love and affection	Not enough time
For the children	Poor housing for pet
Someone to greet me	Location dangerous for pet
Property protection	Pets not allowed
Someone to care for	Family allergy problems
Beauty of animal	Dislike animals
Sport (e.g. hunting)	Too expensive
Show value	Zoonoses

may often be flawed by the methods of delivery and the type of respondent. Nevertheless, the results are broadly similar, with dogs and cats usually being kept for companionship. Dogs may also be owned for protection and for sporting or work reasons (Table 7.4). For instance, in some countries dogs are kept for work rather than companionship, and in Taiwan more people keep a dog for protection (47%) than for companionship (41%) (Hsu *et al.*, 2003). Also, many people have a pet to act as a confidante and source of emotional support for their children (Kidd *et al.*, 1992), but this is often misguided and dogs are sometimes returned to shelters because they fail in these areas (Phipps, 2003). Pre-adolescents reported that their families acquired a pet because of a 'pet-deficit', a perception that a pet was needed to complete the environment of a normal family (Davis, 1987). It is evident that the major reasons for owning pets are owner-focused and may not reflect the needs of the animal (Table 7.4). Yet, interestingly, those who choose not to have a pet do so primarily for reasons relating to the possibility of there being problems with its welfare.

7.4.2 The human–companion animal bond reflects attachments and benefits in both directions

The nature of the human–companion animal bond has been investigated using a range of measures described in detail by Anderson (2007). This is not attitudinal research; rather, it attempts to quantify the strength of the bond between humans and companion animals usually by assessing attachment, but also by evaluating abuse and neglect. However, although the results relate the strength of bond between human and dog, for instance, they do not present any biological perspective on this relationship. The strength or weakness of such bonds may be reflected in similar relationships in other societies between people and cattle or people and pigs, but these bonds have not been quantified.

The domestication of the wolf and subsequent evolution of the dog through natural and artificial selection has produced an animal adapted to a human environment. This attachment of dogs to people may be quantified using techniques developed to assess the attachment of children to adults such as the 'strange situation test'. Dogs were found to have a clear preference for their owners than for others, a result which indicates a clear attachment for specific humans. In addition, dogs may have evolved abilities to pick out specific acoustic clues and use them in relation to the environment. Humans, even those without dogs, can understand the meaning of different dog barks, suggesting that dogs have evolved vocal behaviour which can be interpreted by humans to the benefit of the dog. Dogs may also respond to human body language (pointing, looking) better than wolves (Miklosi *et al.*, 2003). This is probably an outcome of domestication as, in addition, goats also are quite adept at responding to human body language (Kaminski *et al.*, 2005).

Studies of the physiological impacts of human-to-dog interactions have tended to focus on human responses but there have also been some important observations on the physiological responses of dog-to-human interactions. Dogs are focused on human activity and are attached to them. When women petted dogs the animals' plasma stress hormone (cortisol) levels were lower than when they were petted by men (Hennessy *et al.*, 1997), and they also showed more relaxed behaviour. Gentle handling by humans also reduced canine blood pressure (Lynch and Gantt, 1968). Thus, at least some features of physiological stress responses and the behaviour of dogs appear to be particularly sensitive to human interactions. Odendaal and Menitjes (2003) found that when people, both owners and non-owners, spoke gently to dogs and petted them that blood pressure decreased in both the people and the dogs. Moreover, there were other changes in plasma levels consistent with calming effects of petting on both. These mutual physiological changes suggest that such social interaction is beneficial to the dog and the human. Although there is little evidence that cats respond physiologically to gentle human interactions, individual cats certainly show behavioural responses to human petting and handling that suggest pleasure.

These observations, combined with those of Hemsworth and Coleman (1998) and their colleagues, suggest that fully domesticated animals are not only confident in the company of humans, but that the presence of humans engaging in gentle interaction with the animals has positive physiological effects and beneficial outcomes. This suggests an extremely important role for human behaviour in the health and welfare of all domesticated animals, as considered further in Chapter 3.

7.4.3 Problems with day-to-day management of companion animals, especially dogs, often revolve around behavioural difficulties

Although the relationship between humans and dogs, and human attitudes towards companion animals or pets, especially dogs, have been investigated in some depth, the day-to-day management of pets has been poorly investigated (Kobelt, 2004). Again, most research has depended on questionnaire studies, with resultant biases, as (1) they are often distributed from veterinary clinics and therefore are only answered by veterinary clients and (2) they are often long and unfriendly and only answered by enthusiasts. Management varies considerably depending on the species of pet and the breed, particularly of dogs. The management requirement in terms of human interaction, exercise, play and work are unknown. Separation anxiety, which affects some dogs and cats, occurs usually when a favoured person is absent. Such anxiety can be severe for some animals. The main risk factor for this condition is living in a home with a single adult; dogs living with one adult are 2.5 times more likely to experience separation anxiety than dogs living in multiple-adult households (Flannigan and Dodman, 2001). This illustrates how the environment a dog inhabits can negatively affect its psychological well-being.

Interestingly, the majority of dog owners report that their animal has a behaviour problem. The problem may range from being a minor nuisance to the owner, such as leaping up on visitors, of little significance to the dog, such as annoying the neighbourhood by barking, or of major consequences for the dog, such as severe anxiety (Stafford, 2006). Anxiety-related disorders are probably the commonest class of problems in pets (Overall, 1997). Abnormal behaviours which reflect anxiety and fear in dogs may include those indicating separation anxiety, phobias and dominance aggression. Stereotypic behaviours or obsessive-compulsive behaviours are also seen in dogs. Dogs with behavioural problems are less likely to be interacted with by their owner and to be exercised and walked in public. The major reason owners give for surrendering their dogs or cats for euthanasia by shelters or pounds is that they engage in an unacceptable behaviour (Overall, 1997).

The study of the aetiology, expression and treatment of behavioural problems in companion animals, especially dogs and cats, is in its infancy. The degree to which appropriate or inappropriate interaction by humans with dogs or cats leads to fear, anxiety or aggression in these animals is unclear. However, the behaviour of pets living in close contact with humans can be easily influenced by human behaviour, so that dogs, for instance, can easily be inadvertently trained to engage in inappropriate behaviour such as mounting or barking. It is believed that human behaviour can encourage or reinforce timid behaviour in dogs and probably also influence anxiety and some types of aggression. Thus, the behavioural responses of humans to pet behaviour may have negative impact on the animal's well-being given that anxiety and timidity are unpleasant experiences for animals. Close gentle interactions without correct training may have negative effects on some anxiety-related behaviour of dogs, and hence their welfare, but it has been shown that spoiling activity directed towards dogs does not necessarily increase the risk of separation anxiety (Flannigan and Dodman, 2001).

The ongoing study of behavioural problems in dogs and cats, and particularly improved understanding of the prevention of such behaviours, will have a positive impact on welfare by reducing the number of animals with anxiety problems and by reducing the number left in isolation because of their behaviour. Companion animals without behaviour problems are likely to be treated better by their owners.

In addition, the number surrendered to shelters and pounds should decrease. There remains a lack of understanding of the aetiology of behaviour problems in dogs and cats despite the fact that diagnostic methodologies and treatments are well developed.

Companion animals are often considered part of the family, and some suffer abuse. It is difficult to quantify the abuse of pets, but it has been investigated by attempting to quantify the proportion of animals presented at veterinary clinics with signs of physical abuse (Munro and Thrusfield, 2001a, 2001b, 2001c, 2001d; Williams *et al.*, 2008). Mental abuse is less clearly defined. Perhaps in dogs, vacillating between giving them excessive attention and none, giving them poor training and preparation for life, and reinforcing unwanted behaviours such as fearful behaviour and aggression, would amount to mental abuse. Mental abuse may be considered to exist in households with too many cats where some have behavioural problems associated with anxiety (Overall, 1997). Chronically anxious dogs and cats are common, and this suggests major deficiencies in our management of these animals.

7.4.4 Managing unwanted companion animals is a major issue of welfare concern

The presence of many unwanted dogs and cats in most countries, both rich and poor, and the presence of shelters run by humanitarian organizations and pounds run by local authorities, suggest that there are major problems in our management of companion animals (see Chapter 6). Being caught as a stray or being an unwanted puppy are probably the two major reasons why dogs are killed in wealthy countries. In such countries, few street dogs are evident because regulations governing their management are enforced. In poorer countries, street dogs are common due to the cost of dog control, but also because some people want to have street dogs for various social and religious reasons. Their existence as street dogs and their lack of management lead to poor welfare. A greater understanding of why people want street dogs and how to improve their management – that is, nutritional and breeding management – would enhance their welfare.

7.4.5 Observing diverse human–dog interactions helps the identification of appropriate human behaviour for securing dog welfare

Understanding the reasons why humans choose to own pets aids the development of codes of practice for companion animals, but much more needs to be known about optimizing human–companion animal interactions and pet management for the welfare of the animals to be optimized. The unwillingness of some owners to allow their beloved pet to be euthanized may compromise the animal's welfare, even when its owners are caring and loving people. Understanding grief and how to cope with death are an important element of the modern human–companion animal relationship (Stewart, 2001).

The study of the use and management of working dogs such as guide dogs for the blind, police dogs, military dogs and farm dogs furthers our understanding of the needs of dogs. Working dogs are useful animals, and the study of interactions between them and their handlers reflects how they value their animals. For example, Lloyd (2004) found the second dog a blind person used was much more likely to be rejected than their first or subsequent dogs because of heightened expectations of the handler. It is a similar situation with police dogs, but it is not clear whether this is the case with pet dogs. Unrealistically high expectations of what a dog can do can also have an impact on whether a dog adopted from a shelter is kept or relinquished (Stafford, 2006). A better understanding of human expectations of their companion animals may help improve attitudes and interactions between them and may directly improve the welfare of the animals.

7.5 Animals in Sport and Entertainment

7.5.1 Human attitudes to animals used in entertainment or sport are highly variable

Little is known about the welfare impact on animals of their use in entertainment and sport. Entertainment animals are found in circuses, zoos and petting farms, and are also used for showing and in obedience and activity trials, for example sheep dogs and hunting trials. Sport animals are used in various types of racing, for example sled-dog and greyhound racing, horse racing, eventing and endurance, and in other sports, such as agility, show jumping and hunting. Although the optimal management and incidence of injuries in racing dogs, such as greyhounds and sled dogs, and horses have been researched, and many of the people involved claim to be caring, little is actually known about their relationship with their animals. As expected, however, general observation reveals a wide spectrum of approaches from strong attachment, consideration and balanced welfare management to harmful over-indulgence or callous indifference towards what the animal may experience when serving these human-centred purposes.

7.5.2 Sport animals are often disposed of when their sport ability deteriorates

Those involved with racing horses or dogs believe that successful animals enjoy racing, and greyhounds certainly run freely when following the lure. However, they sustain injuries, particularly to the musculoskeletal system, such as fractures of the carpal and tarsal bones. Racetrack design and the characteristics of the running surface influence both the speed of racing and the type of injuries sustained. A greyhound gets injured on average about once in 25 races (Stafford, 2006), which has significant welfare implications. Moreover, greyhounds usually finish racing at about 3.5 years of age, after which most are killed, and only a small proportion are retained for breeding. This suggests that many people who race greyhounds regard them as of value for only a small part of the animal's potential life. Although increasing numbers of greyhounds are now being adopted as pets after their racing life is over (60% in the USA), this probably does not represent a significant attitudinal change by owners. Rather, it is a response to embarrassment caused by public recognition that large numbers of healthy animals were being killed at very young ages. Indeed, most greyhound owners appear to regard their animals as disposable once their human-centred purpose has been served. Of course, greyhound racing is a commercial activity, via gambling, and economic constraints do not allow those involved in the industry to keep the dogs for their entire lives. Racehorse owners may have similar economic constraints and attitudes to their animals, but little research has been done on this.

Sled-dog racing is less commercial, yet dogs are still required to pull sleds in sprint, long-distance or stage races (Stafford, 2006). Much of the racing is done in very cold conditions and in some cases dogs cover 160 km per day for 8 days or more. This is extremely arduous and metabolically demanding. In the Iditarod race in Alaska, up to a third of dogs do not finish the race because of fatigue, injury, lameness or diarrhoea. Such racing sports, which humans obviously enjoy, use animals at their extreme physical limits and they often become stressed and injured. However, even in less physically demanding sports such as agility trials, dogs may show signs of stress and become highly agitated before competitions (Stafford, 2006). Successful animals obviously cope with the situation in which they are used, but the effects of training and competition on the unsuccessful animals are unknown. Knowledge of the physiology of exercise, responsibly applied, may help to optimize the performance of sports animals while improving their welfare.

7.5.3 Show animals are often bred to have exaggerated non-functional physical characteristics that give expression to the breeders' aesthetic preferences

Animals in entertainment include animals used for showing. Breeding of show animals usually focuses on physical features that conform to specific breed standards and meet the judging requirements (see Chapter 4). This results in show animals, especially dogs but also horses and cats, having extreme physical characteristics which may compromise their welfare (McGreevy and Nicholas, 1999). Moreover, these extreme features are often non-functional, being determined principally by the aesthetic preferences of the breeder. As such, the attitudes of people who breed show animals differ markedly from those whose interest in animals is primarily functional. Indeed, the breeding of such show animals might even be regarded as a living form of artistic expression. However, little research has been carried out on the attitudes of people who show animals.

Environmental Enrichment

Studying the Nature of Nurture

8.1 Environmental Enrichment

Environmental enrichment developed as a topic within animal welfare science around 1980 (Mellen and MacPhee, 2001). It is sometimes described as coming into existence at this time (Chamove, 1994), and many reviews of the subject contain little or no earlier information (Purves, 1997). Environmental enrichment research is, broadly speaking, the study of how the quality of an animal's housing conditions can affect its health, development and well-being.

The term environmental enrichment became a nexus for information-sharing and joint activities, particularly within the zoo-keeping community. Enrichment was adopted as the rallying cry for a grassroots response to the suffering of animals kept under clearly inadequate and often antiquated conditions in many zoological gardens. The concept spread rapidly to laboratories and animal shelters, not only because the animals were kept in similar conditions but also because they were cared for by a similar group of professionals. Shelter staff, animal technicians and zookeepers share many qualities in being typically well educated, highly interested in and compassionate towards animals, and spending extended periods of time in close proximity with animals in the course of carrying out husbandry tasks.

8.1.1 The backlash against 'enrichment' as a scientific concept

The initial burst of applied enrichment research was inventive, enthusiastic and widely discussed. The involvement of research specialists was initially relatively minor, leading to a predominance of work that was anecdotal, unsystematic and lacking a formal theoretical framework. However, some limitations in experimental design were also unavoidable consequences of the applied setting. For example, in zoos there are typically only one or a few animals of each type, and the keepers are motivated to provide maximum, immediate benefit for animals in distress rather than carry out careful examinations of abstract variables.

By the 1990s more empirical grounding and structured theoretical discussion were evident. These coincided with the expansion of formal training for animal technicians in Canada and the USA, and the first systematic meetings and dedicated trade publications focusing on the welfare of these animals, some explicitly using enrichment as a rallying point; for example, the *Shape of Enrichment Newsletter* in 1992 and the First International Conference on Environmental Enrichment in 1993. Like many other scientific notions, for example stress and animal welfare, enrichment emerged from research and was parleyed into a more general social movement and then began to reinsert itself into experimental endeavours in a somewhat different form and with greater urgency. There was an uneasy equilibrium between the semantic weight of social 'buy-in' and the dispassionate precision of scientific enquiry, and a need to maintain a connection between the two.

This research revival provoked some prominent researchers to criticize environmental enrichment as a scientific concept, and to attempt to steer it towards a firmer footing or dispense with it altogether. For instance, Ian Duncan and Anna Olsson (2001) wrote a presentation called *Environmental Enrichment: from flawed concept to pseudo-science* in which they proposed that this concept had been 'adopted by animal welfare science in an uncritical way that is liable to bring this discipline into disrepute.' Ruth Newberry (1995) stated that '...the primary problem is a lack of general theoretical framework for environmental enrichment.' Newberry (1995) and Arnold Chamove (1989) both attempted to provide a uniting theoretical framework of improved biological function or the psychological perception of spaciousness.

It must be noted, however, that environmental enrichment is not just a subset of animal welfare science; it is a fundamental concept that cuts across many disciplines. Research has been carried out under this name actively and continuously since the 1920s. Enrichment research is part of a continuity of research that blends with other interests relating to inputs such as touch, novelty and stress, and outputs such as fear, intelligence and curiosity, none of which can be reliably disentangled and separated (e.g. Renner and Rosenzweig, 1987).

Enrichment also embodies great societal hopes, often in conflicting ways. For example, in the late 1950s and 1960s enrichment studies demonstrated the destructive effects of raising infants in barren isolation. This line of evidence was used to support often conflicting claims; for instance, both that individuals could be provided with conditions that allow them to overcome early childhood disadvantages (Curtis and Nelson, 2003) and that infants raised by the 'incorrect' types of parent were doomed to be irreversibly violent and anti-social (e.g. Harlow, 1959). Enrichment research provides information that is easily embroidered upon, and even distorted, to serve the current aspirations of society; concern for the welfare of captive animals is only the most recent example. In fact, enrichment as a word applies more directly to the current social concern, in this case relating to animal suffering, than to the underlying empirical evidence.

Environmental enrichment is not a superficial idea that animal welfare scientists can easily dispense with or redirect. Rather, it is a more deeply embedded guiding concept which has evolved through sporadic updates and changes of focus, a concept which animal welfare scientists may beneficially explore in order to seek a better understanding of the needs of animals. Study of the history and contemporary uses of the term 'enrichment' can reveal how this concept has, and does, fill numerous roles for many different groups. It certainly behoves animal welfare scientists, as servants of the specific societal concern of 'animal welfare', to understand the origins of this notion and where it might be leading. If they do not choose to participate in its further development, then others are likely to continue without them. If they do take part, a degree of ambiguity and diversity of approach must be tolerated and accommodated if it moves thinking, at least generally, in directions that may be fruitful.

8.1.2 The momentum of enrichment as a research key word

Staff whose primary duty is to work at the cagefront are still likely to have had limited exposure to any experimentally based, hypothesis-driven approaches, and, in many cases, their first duty is to carry out routine husbandry and health care activities. When an enrichment study is carried out the scientific aspect may be compromised either by necessity or through limitations of training and other resources. There is a broad awareness that the animal's interests may not be served by the use of enrichments without specific proven benefits, and often a lack of any benefits at all. This is especially so if these off-target efforts encourage misleading 'window dressing' and complacency.

Conversely, the good of a specific animal is often better served by providing any available interventions that might be beneficial on a precautionary basis, even if, as may often be the case, the positive effects are due largely to a fortuitous impact of novelty and the increased human contact and attention associated with the enrichment programme (Young, 2003). In many facilities breaking the status quo by any means available has been a worthwhile first step. If there is to be a good second step it should involve an appropriate type and degree of scientific involvement.

However, is the best way to take part in this second step to vehemently criticize what has gone before and try to redefine the issue rather than simply improve its focus? It is important that scientists try to 'capture' and perhaps refine the notion of enrichment rather than extinguish or abduct it for their own purposes. This kind of subversion of intent should be familiar to welfare scientists with a feelings focus; they have seen attempts to define welfare in terms that exclude suffering, attempts which were not only undertaken by vested interests but also by other researchers who naturally emphasized the indices they excelled in measuring; for example, fisheries: (Arlinghaus *et al.*, 2007).

Scientists engaging with enrichment must grapple with language that eludes proper definition and approaches that are flawed, and with intuitively developed enrichments which may not always have authenticated effectiveness. But in many cases they *are* effective, and merely lack opportunities to enter the peer-reviewed scientific literature. Animal welfare scientists who are engaged in the area may have a chance to intervene and demonstrate the advances that have been made by practitioners, as well as to, tactfully, illuminate the dead ends entered into. Case studies and epidemiological approaches may have particular value in areas where subjects of each species are few and scattered (Swaisgood and Shepherdson, 2005).

If this endeavour is not constructively embraced it may be removed from professional researchers by the animal-caretaking professionals who are now increasingly trained as scientists in their own right, working in their own manner, which may exclude elements of rigour that it would be preferable to retain. Precisely what would be lost if this were to occur? It is not entirely certain that anything would be lost in that both contenders are largely attempting to invent the field from scratch. But scientists from an academic, inter-disciplinary tradition *should* be better able to place enrichment in its full context of prior research and theory and create a more informed and purposeful line of research with a minimum of unnecessary duplication, while also necessarily appreciating the goals of the industry stakeholders and animal advocates.

There are three particularly productive areas of theory from which to draw. First, there are many psychological theories, generated largely during the mid-1900s, which were developed from studies into critical periods, sensory perception and the effect of the environment upon development. Second, there are historical and contemporary theories relating to physical mechanisms, particularly in the area of neurobiology. Third, there are applied techniques developed to occupy exhibit animals, best represented by the work of Hal Markowitz (e.g. Markowitz, 1982; Markowitz *et al.*, 1990; Markowitz and Aday, 1998). However, the task now is not so much to decide which of these is the most scientifically correct, but to develop a fresh context for the productive use of each and to identify common features. Animal welfare scientists do not need to fill a theoretical void with their own *ad hoc* structures; they may instead excavate, adapt and employ the thoroughly tested structures that already exist but which have fallen into disuse or failed to cross discipline boundaries.

8.2 History

8.2.1 Psychology: how animals change in response to experience

Earlier psychological research, by contrast with the applied zoological setting, employed large groups of uniformly housed rats whose well-being was not a significant consideration. In fact, one reason for building bridges between academic research and animal caretakers might be to curb those excesses in research that have enduringly tarnished the reputation of experimental psychology. Rodent-based research was a standard in many fields of psychology by the middle of the last century, and from this research we have developed an array of tools, including many standardized behaviour tests (see Chapter 6) – for example, open-field tests, mazes and operant procedures – and a body of assumptions including the belief that barren environments create animals which are more fearful and less intelligent than animals kept in less barren environments. These findings have had widespread implications for our treatment of animals and humans.

The first common assertion is that barren environments cause fearfulness. This is often measured as a tendency to *freeze*, or become immobile. But the data in relation to fearful freezing are far less conclusive than might be assumed. Although early experiments apparently demonstrated that rats from barren environments are less active in a novel enclosure, this is often not the case or they are more active (e.g. Ader, 1965; Gill *et al.*, 1966; Holson, 1986; but see Denenberg and Morton 1962; Brown, 1968; Smith, 1972; Morgan, 1973). The reasons for this and other inconsistencies have never been properly examined, but there are some potential culprits as yet not commented upon. For example, the shorter the duration of the test the more likely it is that the predicted relationship will be found. Moreover, it is known that the relationship between housing and activity vanishes unless the open field is the first test performed, which suggests that any effect is transient and erodes rapidly across a few days of testing or even within the few minutes of the test itself.

The second common assertion is that barren housing reduces intelligence. Within one recent peer-reviewed paper, animal research supporting this proposition was referred to as 'very consistent' producing 'invariably, similar results' that demanded an explanation for the failure of downstream initiatives to increase human IQ in pre-schoolers (Curtis and Nelson, 2003). However, the findings in animals were never as unanimous or convincing as they have been painted.

The intelligence of rats was typically measured in mazes, with those from more barren environments taking longer to traverse and entering more blind alleys on the way to their reward, than those from less barren environements. However, early research established that the 'impaired' rats could perform as well as those from enriched cages if more highly motivated by greater hunger or an electrified floor (Woods *et al.*, 1961). Also, an intervention as limited and simple as providing visual images improved their performance (Walk, 1958). The maze would be a more novel environment to animals from deprived housing; the animals would also have underdeveloped sensory systems and be less physically fit and physically coordinated (see Hymovitch, 1952; Brown, 1968; Kolb and Elliot, 1987). There is no convincing evidence that the disadvantage demonstrated in maze tests is entirely, or even predominantly, cognitive.

Subsequent data using other methods such a T-maze, the Lashley jumping stand and operant responding have not found a gross cognitive deficit in animals from barren environments. For example, discrimination learning is not typically impaired (Bingham and Griffiths, 1952; Gill *et al.*, 1966) and impaired discrimination reversal is only sometimes found.

Rats from barren environments experienced greater frustration: they responded more when rewards were withdrawn, rather like an annoyed customer kicking the broken vending machine, and this interfered with their ability to demonstrate learning (Davenport *et al.*, 1976; Woodcock, 2004). Moreover, they responded at high rates when low rates would earn more rewards, and they could be slow to change behaviour to meet new reinforcement contingencies (Morgan, 1973). They showed higher, quicker, operant-response rates for food (Rose, 1988), and showed higher operant demand for food. It may also be true that aversive stimuli, such as shock, are more aversive to rats from barren housing as they significantly outperformed enriched rats on a shock-avoidance task (Parsons and Spear, 1972). Operant techniques are available to control for these factors. When they were employed, cognitive differences between enriched and deprived rats were difficult to find, and in some cases deprived animals outperformed those from enriched caging, perhaps due to their greater motivation for food (Patterson-Kane, 1999).

However, theoretical researchers are generally more interested in using the open field and maze as a tool than questioning their validity, while animal welfare researchers are more enthusiastic about demonstrating deficits produced by poor housing than questioning whether or not deficits exist. In animal welfare science, negative findings of this type not only elicit reduced interest but also generate greater scepticism about one's ethical motivation for somehow generating this currently counter-intuitive outcome.

Psychology experiments between the 1920s and 1970s were preoccupied with how experiences during the juvenile period affected an animal's later abilities. The driving force of this experimentation was a concern with parenting, creating functional citizens and understanding the fundamental adaptive capacities of the individual. However, the implicit presupposition in much of this work was that early-life experiences had important long-term consequences. Researchers were therefore predisposed to conform their findings to these expectations, much as some/many animal welfare researchers are currently predisposed to find that enrichment improves all aspects of animal welfare. Thus, despite the mixed findings, general mechanisms were proposed to link enriched conditions with enhanced performance, often giving little or no attention to contrary and missing evidence.

The mechanisms proposed fall into two basic areas of 'transfer' and 'emotional immunization'. Transfer theories suggest that animals cope poorly with entirely novel experiences, so the broader range of experiences in the enriched cage produces animals better able to cope with similar challenges later in life by being less fearful and/or having better understanding (e.g. Zimbardo and Montgomery, 1957; Soskin, 1963; Benefiel and Greenough, 1998). Emotional immunization is a concept which extends this notion by suggesting that animals with broad experience cope better even with purely novel situations for which they have previously learned no specific coping skills; they also become more actively exploratory and stimulus-seeking (e.g. Levine, 1960; Einon and Morgan, 1976; Rose et al., 1987), whereas animals from deprived environments become passive and fearful (Wemelsfelder, 1997b).

Although learning is mentioned and assessed, psychological theories tended to emphasize emotional competence, boldness or arousal. More recent conceptions of this general idea suggest a shift in an animal's optimal level of arousal so that animals from barren environments become stressed under levels of stimulation where enriched animals are still exploratory and able to learn effectively. However, in rats this difference is often relatively fleeting and soon extinguished by improved housing, handling or testing.

8.2.2 Neurology: how inadequate environments damage animals

Neurologists pioneered the rat as a scientific model, and there has been consistent study for over a hundred years into the physical effects of enrichment. The basis for this is easy to understand; when picking up rats from differential housing those from barren and enriched conditions not only behave differently they also look different and *feel* markedly different in your hand. It is therefore apparent in these terms that there are gross physical consequences of different housing conditions. Interestingly, the first reported enrichment study preceded the modern era by at least a century and a half, and was concerned with effects on the brain. In 1791, Malacarne demonstrated that birds taught to sing had more convoluted brain structures than did other birds (as described by Rosenzweig et al., 1972).

With rats, during the middle of the last century enrichment research was spearheaded by the University of California Berkeley group who demonstrated extreme and widespread differences in brain size, anatomy and neurochemistry (reviewed in Renner and Rosenzweig, 1987; Young, 2003). Hebb (1949) initially suggested that stimulation caused firing of cells in the brain and strengthened connections between them. This speculation was supported by finding wide-ranging deficits, including increased dendritic arborization and neurogenesis (e.g. Holloway, 1966; Kempermann et al., 1997). Although a connection is easily assumed to exist there is, in fact, no clear correspondence between these neurological findings and behavioural competence. Specifically, attempts to connect arborization with performance on cognitive tests have been negative (e.g. Anderson, 1995), and other data showed that differences in brain mass could occur due to a range of impositions, in each case *without* impairing cognitive performance; for example, a 7% loss of weight due to the effect of a toxins (Ferguson *et al.*, 1993) compared with the 7–8% difference found in enrichment studies (e.g. Rosenzweig *et al.*, 1972).

Researchers with a neurobiological emphasis tended to frame the same syndrome of behavioural responses observed by psychologists in terms of cognition – that is, learning and memory – rather than emotion. Enrichment was seen as providing learning opportunities (e.g. Rosenzweig and Bennett, 1972). Thus, it is not sufficient for the environment to be stimulating; it must also present satisfying consequences contingent upon learned behaviours.

The finding of brain impairment revealed by the neurobiological-cognitive approach has important implications for animal welfare thinking. Behaviour is context-specific, so that boldness will help a rat find food one day and make it *become* food for a predator another. Whereas behaviour usually has a meaning in terms of its function it only rarely has an indisputable 'goodness' or 'badness'. What was important was not that the neurological underdevelopment caused by barren environments was severe and irreversible (that, incidentally, has not been comprehensively shown), it was that it occurred at all. This showed that the animal kept in barren housing was demonstrably impaired and defective, not just different or adapted to a specific environment. This orientation provided a fresh focus for animal welfare investigations as it suggested that the relevant independent variable was not *enrichment*, but environmental *impoverishment*, where enriched conditions helped to produce development that more greatly exploited the animal's potential.

These observations are naturally of great concern to researchers attempting to provide normal animals of use in species conservation or as biomedical models. Neurological deficits create a compelling connection between effective enrichment, skilled husbandry and valid science. Yet, it is only recently that this concern has begun to penetrate the biomedical community at large, and this has arisen mainly through neurobiological research rather than research with a predominantly animal welfare focus. For example, it has been noted that many genetically abnormal or modified animals displayed untoward symptoms only when kept under barren housing conditions (e.g. Spires *et al.*, 2004). It has even been suggested that to effectively phenotype new mutant rodents they must be observed in a naturalistic home-cage (van der Staay and Steckler, 2002), rendering the laboratory animal more like a zoological exhibit than a domesticated animal. There is a slow-dawning realization that animals in barren environments may not be valid models for human conditions that arise in relatively normal environments due to specific congenital vulnerabilities and/or environmental insults. The laboratory animal's environment should be abnormal only to the extent that the abnormality is a planned factor contributing to the model.

8.2.3 Subjective experience: occupations for animals in zoos

Unfortunately, much of the applied enrichment work in zoos that has been conducted in the field is either undocumented or difficult to locate (Young, 2003). One prominent exception is the work by Markowitz (1982) with animals which had been kept, long-term, in barren zoo environments. The focus in these cases was upon providing the animals with something that occupied their attention. Markowitz developed operant methods to produce engineered mechanisms that responded to the animal's behaviour. The use of such mechanisms also developed into the use of overt training. This approach has been developed, or in many cases re-invented, in zoo-based initiatives to promote natural behaviour through training, devices and novel stimuli (e.g. Young, 2003; see also the annual International Conferences On Environmental Enrichment, 1993–2005)

This emphasis on allowing animals to perform behaviours with consequences and exercise some control over the environment marries well with the neurobiological emphasis on opportunities to learn and develop understanding of the environment. However, the motivation in this case is more consistent with psychological theories associated with providing appropriate levels of stimulation and allowing animals to experience positive states of arousal associated with goal-directed behaviour.

Grassroots efforts at enrichment can be found in trade journals such as *The Shape of Enrichment*, which place an emphasis on the working animal caretaker's efforts to improve the lives of their charges, often through knowing the animal and by trial and error rather than the experimental method.

8.3 Mechanism

8.3.1 Harm, enjoyment and the need for environmental contingencies

The need, overall, for environmentally positive, negative and/or challenging, but largely conquerable, features is a core agreed theory underlying all enrichment research. The experimental data show that animals require long-term, meaningful and appropriate stimulation to develop all of their underlying physical systems and to express normal behaviour. Different competencies require different experiences to develop, and impairment may be long-lasting or even permanent with animals that have restricted sensitive periods during development. The type of stimulation required on one level is bemusingly complex and encompasses a range of species-specific requirements. On another level it is also fairly simple in that an approximation of the natural conditions is normally sufficient. Research is required largely in the area of making substitutions for environmental features that are impossible, or deemed too costly, to reproduce. However, once an animal has become impaired its environmental requirements will be altered, either for a limited period of adjustment or permanently. Thus, such abnormal animals may require abnormal environments to experience their best possible subjective welfare.

Applied studies show evidence that moving normal animals into barren conditions can also produce immediate emotional experiences of frustration, fear, aggression, boredom or stress, with resultant immediate injuries. These acute effects will also show rapid improvement when the deficit is corrected. In many cases, there will be abnormalities in both the animals and the environment, yet corrective modifications may need to restrict naturalistic normality, for example escape, sexual or aggressive behaviour, in order to accommodate human use, such as exhibition and handling. For these reasons researchers should be free to employ whichever theoretical concept is most relevant to the situation at hand. Even within the same facility animals will have radically different needs.

A common finding across all areas is that the most effective enrichments are those that create a reasonable approximation to what is natural for the species; that is, conditions that allow the animal's behaviour to have satisfying consequences. For example, juvenile rodents provided with nesting material rapidly developed the ability to build nests that they could use to regulate their exposure to light, cold and aggression. If they were not provided with this material until they were adults their ability to manipulate it to form a functional nest was impaired and often entirely absent. This nesting material allowed the animal to develop a competency, exhibit normal behaviour and experience satisfying outcomes (Van Loo and Baumans, 2004). The provision of nesting material to rodents which are already adult will lead, and has led, to the conclusion that rats do not build nests and thus do not require nesting material. Also, if rodents become competent nest-builders disruption of this behaviour can provide a simple and broadly sensitive test of impairments of phenotype (Deacon, 2006).

8.3.2 Apocryphal mechanisms: explanations should match data

The fact that barren environments cause neurobiological harm to animals is an important component of the overall picture. However, there has always been a tendency to reach for a 'hard science' mechanistic explanation in experiments in other domains. Pioneers of the field such as Hebb and Pavlov routinely speculated about the underlying neurology when their only direct recordings were of behaviour and bodily processes outside the brain. In reaching beyond the data, there is always a danger of using an explanation from the wrong domain, or incorrectly generalizing from one to another.

Let us consider the study of the so-called Mozart effect. The assertion that music can increase human intelligence is based on a very small data set in three areas, as follows: (1) a few experiments found that human adults listening to Mozart performed better, specifically on spatial learning tasks performed immediately afterwards (e.g. Rauscher et al., 1995); (2) human children who were taught to play a musical instrument might experience advantages in other areas of learning (Rauscher and Zupan, 2000); and (3) rats raised in cages subject to the playing of Mozart, compared with silence or its perceptual equivalents, performed better on mazes (Rauscher et al., 1998).

On this basis it was proposed that the effect was due to melodic content, relied upon cognition and had a neural basis. Music may in fact have complex cognitive and neurological effects, but the onus should be on the research to demonstrate them convincingly, which it has not yet done, before popularizing the concept to the extent that fetal or newborn human infants are being bombarded with classical music in the womb or crib. It is also crucial to draw attention to the fact that all of the existing data with rats, including studies on music, relate to the effects of raising animals in destructive subnormal environments and not to putative enhancements in normal environments.

8.4 Rethinking Enrichment

There are a plethora of specific theoretical contexts of relevance to enrichment, ranging from Freudian psychology to neurobiology. But the general consensus is that barren environments over long periods produce animals with impaired coping abilities, and over short periods they produce negative mental states relating to lack of opportunity to perform behaviours with satisfying consequences.

There is further evidence that both the emotional and physical harms caused by barren environments are remarkably reversible in rats and somewhat reversible in many species. It must also be acknowledged that all of the data so far are subject to serious confounding variables. In behavioural data, fearfulness impaired a wide battery of cognitive tests and *physical exercise alone* had a similar degree of neurobiological effect (e.g. Brown *et al.*, 2003). Even with neurobiological and related sciences the concept of enrichment is more a matter of aspiration than hard data. The true effects of enrichment depend heavily on many factors that have not been systematically varied in our over-dependence both upon a rat model and upon a few poorly validated behavioural tests.

It must also be noted that the judgement that fearfulness is negative *per se* applies safely only to domesticated animals, as wild animals often need to be highly averse to novel, potentially harmful stimuli which may prove to be predators, competitors, toxins and other hazards. It is partly for this reason that captive-raised animals survive poorly in the wild (e.g. Jule *et al.*, 2008). Rats raised in enriched housing were apparently at increased initial risk of predation compared with those from barren cages (Roeder *et al.*, 1980). Primates raised without mothers were less aggressive, but in the wild higher levels of aggression were crucial for developing normal social relations (Chamove *et al.*, 1984). With domesticated livestock, humans tend initially to be treated as predators and sometimes with aggression, but these normal 'wild' behaviours will have net negative outcomes in closely managed circumstances and so are discouraged (see Chapter 7). Likewise, laboratory animals must submit to procedures, including human handling, and many zoo animals require a degree of veterinary monitoring and movement between areas. So an ideal rearing environment for such animals will depend upon our scientifically informed views on how they should live, tempered by complex levels of ethical judgement. In reality, however, some trade-offs are made to accommodate the primary uses to which we put the animals in different categories.

Historical data demonstrate that barren housing causes neurobiological deficits and modifies behavioural responsiveness. When considering how environments have modified an animal and its chronic behavioural tendencies the crucial concepts seem to be brain impairment and emotional arousal. It is clear that delivery of any enrichment should identify specific deficits and attempt to treat those rather than aim for some poorly defined global improvement by adding whatever feature takes our human fancy. There is also strong evidence that enrichment should not attempt to be maximally stimulating, especially when animals have a lower tolerance for novelty and change. In fact, the first consideration should probably be to provide secure shelter areas which allow the animals to retreat.

Applied work has typically not focused on identifying damage to animals and treating it, or supporting the special needs that captivity may create. Instead, the emphasis has been on the animal's acute mental state and current behaviour. The behaviour of animals being exhibited is typically very passive although it may also include overt abnormalities, for example stereotypies. Animals are correspondingly seen as experiencing levels of boredom or frustration that are in need of alleviation. This is highly consistent with animal welfare science where welfare is understood largely in terms of negative subjective experiences (Chapters 1 and 5).

Despite its enduring utility and continuous history, environmental enrichment does have problematical aspects. Enrichment has always implied that we are 'adding to' or 'enhancing' the environment (see Mellen and MacPhee, 2001) and causing an 'increase in functional efficiency' of the animal (Rose, 1988). A 'harm' perspective focuses on the fact that captive environments are damaging animals. It is not for us to decide what we might like to add to the environment, but to identify what present and absent features are causing harm, and to correct them. Much as captive populations may at best preserve as much as possible of a population's genetic diversity while inevitably losing some proportion of it, captive environments must strive to support the best possible development of physical and behavioural systems and an understanding that a degree of untapped potential is bound to remain.

8.4.1 Concept interactions: enrichment for welfare, standardization for science, pragmatism in industry

To this point criticisms of enrichment have focused on its poor performance as a scientific concept. These are valid to the extent that enrichment is embraced at the level of hypothesis formation. In applied settings, however, enrichment is more appropriately a statement of aspiration and a general semantic category, and should be criticized only to the extent that it represents an invalid goal.

Enrichment as a goal is imperfect but it is also powerful and necessary. Its role might include counterbalancing the great scientific weight placed on standardization through minimization. Standardization is a useful goal but is often pursued at the expense of external validity and animal welfare, through omitting every feature of the environment not known to be crucial for life. Moreover, it is commonly adhered to as a doctrine for its own sake, often without regard to the requirements of a specific situation. A precautionary approach to standardization as a primary goal led Bantin and Sanders (1989) to say that we should do nothing unless animals are 'proven to suffer by our practices'. Another approach would be to make our best approximation of a good environment as a starting point (e.g. Stricklin, 1995). Enrichment is one way of encapsulating this alternative perspective by asserting the naturalistic or ethologically designed environment as standard.

However, the two issues of enrichment and standardization should not be seen as entirely in opposition. For example, enrichment research would in many cases benefit from greater standardization just as standard practices would benefit from being more ethologically sound. One of the ongoing problems with drawing conclusions from so-called standardized behavioural tests that provide the basis of what we consider to be the fundamental benefits of enriched environments is that they have not been standardized at all. As Walsh and Cummins (1976) wrote of the open-field test, 'almost every physical characteristic of the apparatus, its surroundings and every procedural step have been widely varied.' The underlying unreliability of many findings within enrichment research arises for two main reasons: insufficient standardization of the behavioural tests, and inappropriate standardization in choosing to rely almost exclusively upon a rat model. Regarding the latter point, it is important to emphasize that the rat's adaptable natural history (as 'vermin') may mean that we are trying to study the destructive effects of poor housing on a species uniquely equipped to resist and rapidly recover from such hardship.

Meanwhile, one of the guiding principles held to by zookeepers, animal technicians and stockpersons is to make do with the limited resources and control available to them for their prescribed duties. This reality has some troubling consequences for both the scientific method and the scope attributed to environmental enrichment.

Kulpa-Eddy et al. (2005) wrote, 'Enrichment conjures images of the fortification of cereal or white bread with vitamins, and implies the addition of ingredients otherwise missing in an impoverished environment.' It is perhaps unavoidable that most workers at the cagefront must try to identify and add specific missing 'vitamins', but considering only what is in the cage not what the cage is. More complex questions are now being asked about how to best keep certain animals, be they laboratory rats or circus elephants, and whether to keep them at all; scientific research should inform these debates. Rather than be critical that enrichment fails in scientific rigour, researchers might raise the issue that enrichment just as frequently fails in its narrow scope because not only do animal welfare scientists often hold it at arms length and with limited acceptance, so also do those in control of grant proposals and budgeting, regulations and guidelines, and facility design at a basic level. Difficult decisions need to be made about just how well we want animals to be kept, and who is going to pay for it on the scale of entire industries from zoo exhibits to battery cages. A plastic toy or puzzle feeder in the cage should not be seen as a typical sort of enrichment for the animal any more than a vitamin tablet should be seen as a meal.

Enriched environments as they were initially conceived included objects chosen relatively arbitrarily that were introduced and regularly changed in order to provide an element of novelty. Later applied research has generally been carried out in contexts where environmental size and fixtures could not be substantially changed, and as a result social groups could also not be radically altered. Accordingly, a great many studies manipulated only the provision of objects and still referred to this single manipulation as enrichment despite evidence that enrichment *per se* exists only as an interaction of many elements (see van Praag *et al.*, 2000). Subsequent studies then found that animals generally lost interest in these objects within minutes or at the most a few days. This led to widespread suggestions that habituation is an issue with enrichment in general, rather than only with aspects relating solely to novelty.

It *must* be remembered that enrichment refers to an entire environment and a substantial change; its use in relation to relatively trivial changes that do not provide meaningful contingencies should be challenged. It is often mentioned that enrichment as a word has a great deal of unfortunate and false implications, such as a 'better than normal state', but it also has some very useful implications of a *full and meaningful improvement*.

Early research was motivated by an ethically neutral desire to understand how physical and behavioural systems within an animal respond to different types of stimulation. As such, enrichment was seen as an improvement relative to the status quo of housing at that time, for example a 20-cm^3 rat cage with a wire mesh floor. It is widely acknowledged that these standard conditions were causing harm to animals, and improvements were moving the animal towards a normal state. Thus, enrichment is a potentially misleading term in suggesting an improvement above the norm. However, calls to replace the term cannot overcome more than a hundred years of use and discontinuing its use makes research inaccessible to those accustomed to employing enrichment as a key word. Pragmatically speaking we can only focus on correcting associated language to avoid terms suggestive of improvement, and emphasize the use of words such as normalize or ameliorate. The enriched condition needs to be seen as a baseline from which deficits are measured. If enrichment is to be replaced it must be by a term that emerges naturally from the verbal community.

8.4.2 What is enrichment good for? (What is it not?)

Enrichment is used both in research and application to suggest the general finding that in order to develop normally and have a good quality of life individuals must live in a satisfactory physical and social environment. There is a long history of interest in what exactly constitutes a good environment, and the mechanism by which a poor environment causes distress and impairment. But empirical progress in both of these areas is slow given the immense complexity of the systems involved. An empirical experiment needs to be conceptualized far more specifically in terms of the actual independent variable, dependent variable and the proposed mechanism (psychological or physical) that connects the two. Ultimately, environmental enrichment does not function as a part of the scientific hypothesis, and it would be clearer to refer to any specific experiment in far more immediately descriptive terms.

Enrichment is a broad semantic category based on an appreciation of the sensitivity of animals to their environments, with the immediate implication that we have an ethical obligation to provide captive animals with well-designed housing, similar to the concept of 'husbandry' with livestock, as distinct from 'animal science'. For this reason enrichment is an excellent theme upon which to base conferences, publications and job descriptions, and it is a reasonable key word to place upon relevant empirical work to facilitate its application. It is already in widespread use with many positive effects on the visibility of the problem and cohesion of efforts to address it. However, environmental enrichment cannot be satisfactorily defined as an independent variable, mechanism of effect or dependent variable, and should not be used in this role.

Theories exist within various sections of enrichment which, at the broadest level, all relate to the effects of the absence of opportunities for constructive, species-appropriate behaviour. Included within these theories are the mediating variables of impaired neurobiological development, the animal's orientation to and emotional response to stimuli, and its immediate emotional states. Researchers should employ the concepts most closely related to their goals, and therefore the variables they are directly measuring, allowing them to work with the concepts' falsifiability. Environmental enrichment is a complex and flawed approach but it has traction, adherents and some sound basic assumptions. Animal welfare scientists might productively contribute to this field, and would also have something to gain from participating in it.

Social Contexts of Animal Welfare

9.1 Animal Welfare is a Human Social Concern

During the 1980s, science began to focus increasingly on the animal's perspective. That is, instead of looking *at* animals with pity or concern it became legitimate to appreciate how the world looked to them. This shift belatedly brought the mainstream scientific view of animal welfare much closer to that of the lay public and, interestingly, provided impetus to the establishment of the now well-recognized discipline of animal welfare science. Empathy-based concerns came to the fore with the empowerment particularly of urban populations and women (e.g. Serpell, 2005), and were also reflected in the rise of humane societies, driven, for instance, by concern for working horses in cities and the treatment of pets.

Acknowledging empathy as the driving force behind welfare concerns leads to the view that an animal that has good welfare is one that is experiencing positive subjective states; that is, overall, it is a contented or happy animal. Or more conservatively, an animal that has uncompromised welfare is one that is not experiencing negative subjective states; that is, an animal that is not suffering (e.g. Brambell, 1965; Duncan, 1981, 2005; Dawkins, 1983, Poole, 1997; Chapters 1 and 5). Essentially, therefore, animal welfare science took on the role of understanding, as best it could, the animal's experience.

9.1.1 Human concern properly relates only to those animals whose welfare we affect

A fuller understanding of our preoccupation with the nature of what animals can experience, which is currently a major focus of animal welfare science, needs to reflect our human ethical concern for the well-being of animals. This ethical concern springs from the existence of reciprocal social relationships with specific animals and an enduring social contract with entire species, such as domesticated animals (see Rollin, 1995). Accordingly, we are representing the animal's point of view only to the extent that there is a human ethical desire to provide a good quality of life to the animals with which we interact.

Our sphere of ethical concern is typically limited to those sentient animals whose welfare we affect by our interactions with them, so that unconstrained wild animals might be excluded. Of course, like domesticated animals, wild animals can obviously also experience suffering and positive states, and are similarly individual, emotional beings. However, if in their natural state they contrive somehow to never encounter human beings or our influence upon their environments these internal states remain entirely the concern of those animals and other non-human animals that they encounter. Domesticated animals have entered into an alliance with the human species. However, as we humans became a dominant superpower species we not only began to have increasingly negative impacts on wild species whose environments we have appropriated, but we also engaged in more uneven and exploitative relationships with domesticated animals which no longer have the option of defection or independence.

Exclusion of the welfare of many wild animals from our sphere of concern does not belittle their capacities. It simply acknowledges that they are independent agents in charge of their own affairs. As Peter Singer (1990) writes: 'We should not try and police all of nature', which is to say, how non-human animal societies deal with each other is in fact none of our concern if we have not made it so by intervening. It follows that our welfare concerns should more properly focus on relations between our own species and those with which we interact, and particularly those we employ or exploit.

9.1.2 Animal welfare scientists mediate between human and non-human societies

In this context, therefore, one role of animal welfare scientists is to consider cases of animal use, by employing our best understanding of the needs of both the human user and the animals themselves, with the relative emphasis between the two being negotiated within ethical frameworks that should be clear and overt. In other words, there is a dual remit: first, to understand and implement the will of the general (human) public regarding the acceptable use of animals, and second, to understand and accommodate the needs of (non-human) animals to live their own lives. As such, animal welfare scientists also tend to act as a conduit between aligned human groups concerned only with being animal advocates and those associated with animal-based industries as enthusiastic producers or consumers; at the same time they attempt to accommodate the needs of the less emphatic, largely detached occupiers of the middle ground (e.g. Schroder and McEachern, 2004). From this perspective, the rigorous methodology of animal welfare science, which involves the 'neutral' language of empirical evidence and rational argument deployed within explicit ethical frameworks, is an invaluable tool as its practitioners engage in this mediating role.

9.1.3 Animal welfare science culture may interfere with this mediating role

As has occurred when other disciplines have emerged, animal welfare science has rapidly become a community and culture in its own right, a development that, in the wider social context, may not be seen as entirely fortunate. Although the development of the discipline has spurred great research, training, funding and discussion of some crucial issues, it has also fostered and perpetuated some specific beliefs. Animal welfare science has become a subset of biology, colonized haphazardly by an amalgam of existing disciplines including nutritional, environmental, health, behavioural and cognitive-neural sciences (Gonyou, 1994; Mellor and Reid, 1994; Chapter 1) and economics. This has implications related to the non-reflective adoption of the specialized languages and particular assumptions of some of these disciplines; for example, relating to death and cognition.

9.1.3.1 Acceptability of death and killing

Euthanasia of animals is in general use and is considered to be an acceptable way of avoiding or ending an animal's suffering. Indeed, many animal welfare scientists would contend that, provided the killing method is humane, no animal welfare compromise occurs. This approach demonstrates a preference for death before discomfort, and possibly also an unwillingness to accept death as a significant event. If this approach is adopted without question it has several implications. First, it would prevent proper consideration of positive welfare, as the potential for future enjoyment is one motivation for supporting continued life. Second, although death *as an abstract concept* is not important to animals, it shares this abstract quality with animal welfare. In contrast, both concepts are highly important to people who carry out the animal-based tasks on a day-to-day basis, including animal care and animal killing. Moreover, killing is often conducted on the assumption that death can be delivered without pain and distress. However, this is difficult to reliably achieve, and offending methods remain in use. There may be greater impetus to re-examine the acceptability of those methods which do cause significant and unnecessary suffering if the acceptability of killing as a strategy were itself to be reconsidered. Death, euthanasia and/or culling methods are largely neglected central concerns of great importance in organic farming (Lund and Olsson, 2005), rehabilitation, laboratory science, pet care and the racing industries. A willingness to kill as a convenience or precaution jars with many people, suggesting a disjunction between those who sanction it and members of the general public; for instance the extensive precautionary foot-and-mouth culling in the UK in 2001 caused widespread criticism even though the animals were in any case ultimately destined for slaughter (Convery *et al.*, 2005).

9.1.3.2 The significance of animal cognition

Some researchers make reference to an animal's cognitive abilities as a yardstick to assess the extent to which they should be concerned about its welfare (e.g. Simmonds, 2006). Mainstream thinking in animal welfare science accepts that many animals have emotions but very few have well-developed cognitive abilities (Dawkins, 1998). Thus, a focus on cognitive ability implicitly means invalidating compassion for many (possibly most) species of non-human animals, as illustrated by the historical arguments of Socrates and Descartes that we need not feel direct moral duties towards animals because they lack reason or language. Yet, extensive data show that many non-human animals can carry out complex feats of learning, memory, categorization and problem-solving, often significantly out-performing humans. A prominent example is Irene Pepperberg's parrot, Alex, which could use abstract concepts including number, colour and material (e.g. Pepperberg, 1987). To argue that high-level cognitive ability is specific to humans and a few privileged species such as apes and cetaceans is to perpetuate an antiquated notion of what such abilities are, which is no less crippling than the denial of non-human animals' emotions. Such marginalization within animal welfare science of issues like cognition may ultimately be just as problematical as the behaviourist prohibition against the scientific study of feelings and thoughts. Moreover, such rejection does not flow inevitably from the central goal of prioritizing animals' emotional states (e.g. Duncan and Petherick, 1991; Mendl and Paul, 2004). However, in saying that basic cognitive competence and the potential for emotional suffering include a wide range of species within the realm of moral consideration, it remains possible that some species may experience particularly egregious forms of negative cognitive and emotional states, such as markedly anxious anticipation of a painful event and protracted grief.

9.2 Sociology Promotes Understanding of Societies and their Interactions

Animal welfare as a human concern arises as much from human behaviour and belief as from our interest in animal experience. The impact of human cultural beliefs must be appreciated in order to understand the reasons given for keeping animals in a certain manner or for mismanaging them when more humane practices are available. In many cases, even without any further research being conducted, more humane alternatives are currently available than are typically in use. Reasons for this include resource constraints and failures of communication. Animal welfare scientists should seek to better understand and exploit the positive beliefs of animal-using groups, and to identify and overcome the bases for resistance to beneficial change.

9.2.1 Human interests: understanding the focus of others will facilitate beneficial change

Most animal-using groups have a positive 'ethic of caring' consistent with their industry and a 'respected body of knowledge' in areas such as experimental use of animals, livestock slaughter and zoo exhibits, which, however, may appear to be more exploitative (see Russow, 2002). An ethic of caring is a basis for a human–animal relationship, and respect for a body of knowledge can indicate openness to new information. However, caring is not the same as animal welfare; it is a method for promoting it, and the related scientific literature, with its objective analytical approach, is often not specifically directed at animal care. Therefore, if we are to be successful in communicating the results of relevant research we must be able to divest ourselves of the trappings of animal welfare 'scientism' and understand the kind of message that will reach particular user groups. As sociologists have been slow to research communities of interest to animal welfare scientists, it is often necessary for such scientists to rely on others who use techniques from their own fields, or on their own observations. This will be illustrated by using examples from research laboratories, agriculture and zoos.

9.2.1.1 Attitudes towards housing of laboratory rats

One example of an area where there is a great deal of research-based information is the housing of rats in the laboratory. Many hundreds of experiments (reviewed by Renner and Rosenzweig, 1987) demonstrated that rats kept in larger cages, in a social group and with nesting facilities are in a superior functional state than those kept alone or in pairs in cages containing only bedding. Yet, typical laboratory housing is barren.

Studies of attitudes of biomedical researchers (e.g. Arluke, 1992) show that there is ongoing resistance to treating animals in the laboratory as sentient individuals, illustrated by taboos on naming or playing with the animals. Attempts to improve animal welfare by challenging such beliefs create a conflict in which the animal user must be proven 'wrong' in their current and traditional practice, so that resistance is evoked and beneficial change is hindered. In addition, standardizing conditions and using valid animal models are important for generating meaningful scientific data. Yet, although data exist which show that current housing does not effectively achieve either goal (e.g. Crabbe *et al.,* 1999; Würbel, 2000), biomedical researchers are often not aware of this despite its importance to them.

However, by changing the focus to improving scientific validity, resistance is often transformed into active solicitation of information. As the goal is to improve the conditions for the animal rather than to spread animal welfare norms, such a change in communication strategy should more effectively reach the scientist whose goal is to optimize the needs of both the animal and animal user. Although it is dispassionately phrased, concern for the validity of the animal model also represents an 'ethic of caring' in that it reflects a desire that the animal should be fully developed and normal in every way. Also, once the animals are placed in the context of a social group and complex environment their behaviour naturally becomes more engaging, and this promotes more effective relationships between investigators and animals, which in turn prompt further concern for animal well-being. For this reason, even small pilot projects should be encouraged as the resulting changes in animal vigour and responsiveness open up avenues for improvement in direct human–animal communication.

9.2.1.2 Attitudes within animal agriculture
In the area of agriculture, animal welfare scientists commonly appear to become aligned more with 'industry' or more as animal advocates. There seems, however, to be much less engagement with farmers as people and as a positive force for change in husbandry conditions. Several studies have shown that farmers are strongly motivated to be effective caretakers of animals (Serpell, 1999). The language of animal welfare tends to be associated with criticism of current practices and judgmental in terms of animal rights, which is alienating and generates resistance (Mellor and Stafford, 2001). However, productive discussions may be started based on concepts of good animal husbandry and stockmanship. In many cases, it will be more productive to make reference to traditional practices rather than recent research results. Farmers are often not highly receptive to discussing concerns about animal suffering and the sentience of individuals (animal point of view, individual) but are highly concerned with filling a role that is protective over the flock or herd

(human point of view, group; Serpell, 1999). In many ways, the focus on welfare at the group level may be more rational than the animal welfare science focus on individuals in a setting where individuals are frequently killed. The focus of animal welfare science on individuals may be at least partly a side effect of many of its practitioners having pet-owning as their main model of human–animal relationships and an associated personal ethic of caring.

9.2.1.3 Constructive approaches in zoos

Zookeepers have a strong focus on 'environmental enrichment' and yet animal welfare scientists addressing them often focus on the inappropriateness of the term and the poor scientific quality of research carried out in this area (see Newberry, 1995; Chapter 8). Rather than expecting workers in zoos to adopt the language and practices of animal welfare science, it might be more productive to present important information in their own terms, and conduct research in collaboration with those expected to implement it. Enrichment is a term that represents the genuine welfare aspiration of the zoological community. Animal welfare scientists should therefore engage with this and attempt to align it to the needs of the animals in exhibits, rather than try to impose their own cultural vocabulary.

9.2.2 Animal societies: the need to be in a group is often underestimated or ignored

It has been acknowledged since antiquity that animals live in societies. Ivar Paulson (1964) suggested that when cultures were based upon hunting there was a deep-seated belief in animal souls, and the need to placate these souls individually and in spiritual aggregates. He suggested, further, that this concern rapidly faded when communities adopted settled agriculture and therefore did not need to be so deeply in tune with animal culture in order to exploit it. In effect, animal culture was once dominant and human species depended upon it. With the advent of widespread domestication the balance of power has been increasingly reversed.

Domesticated species exist most naturally as aggregates. Social bonds are one of the great commonalities between us and many other animal species, including experiences such as social buffering of fear, aggression, care of young and grief. Domesticated animals are derived almost entirely from species that live their entire life in social groups (Chapter 7), and some must be considered almost exclusively at the group level. For example, when Ron Kilgour (1971) was examining and comparing maze performance of various species of animal he discovered that groups of four or five sheep performed better than one sheep alone. It may, in fact, be a vital feature for domesticating many species that they choose to flock together when threatened rather than scatter. It is this social cohesion that supports important processes such as herding, driving and grazing on open pasture.

Thus, to acknowledge that a specific animal is part of our human society only presents some of the picture. Each animal is, or experiences some motivation to be, a member of an own-species community. Accordingly, it is argued here that appropriate handling of most domesticated animals requires not only giving them an appropriate role in our society, but also allowing them to fill an appropriate role in their own society. Our persistent tendency to keep group animals isolated individually, for example pets, some laboratory animals and stable horses, demonstrates an inability to appreciate that they cannot be fully functional in isolation. Research continues to demonstrate the prime importance of social housing.

9.2.3 Animals as subjugated species are disempowered and require advocates

It is particularly the case with large agricultural animals that if the social interactions between and within species are not managed well, and if the animal chooses to withhold cooperation, the human caretaker is placed in a frustrating or even dangerous position. The process of domestication provides a tool to solicit cooperation but it is constrained by the animal being given sufficient motivation and reward to overcome any imposition associated with our use of it. However, technology has increasingly allowed us to bypass cooperative systems and enforce the animal's availability to our will. To highlight this point, it is argued here that driving the imbalance in our relationship to extremes, for purposes other than good caretaking, justifies describing the animals so treated as an 'oppressed group'.

A worrying human habit of subverting the evolved autonomy of animals to our own ends can be seen in many situations. For instance, the solitary pet is left socially and materially dependent on its human caretaker, and artificial insemination of female livestock eliminates the behavioural role of males in that process. This trend is exacerbated by reducing the power of animals in other ways, such as breeding miniaturized species and vulnerable ultra pets (hairless, short-legged, etc.), and removing natural weapons either by breeding (e.g. polled cattle) or amputation (e.g. dehorning and tooth clipping). Such technological adjustments first isolate and then disempower the animals, thereby preventing them from withholding cooperation. This demands that we not only honour but also reinforce our reciprocal social contract with animals, which is that in using them for our purposes, not theirs, we must do so humanely.

Another dimension of human behaviour highlights the need to reinforce our social contract with animals. By deliberately producing powerless individuals we are inevitably producing a group that is more vulnerable not only to exploitation but also to abuse. Given that, at present, there are almost no avenues for many animals to exercise counter-control and so maintain some degree of mutual benefit or minimized abuse they must rely solely on human intervention on their behalf. Thus, animals need human advocates to indicate when exploitation is too severe or insufficiently justified, and they also need human interpreters, including animal welfare scientists, to clarify and convey what animals' needs are and what animals want. Some animal advocates are criticized as not being in tune with economic realities and pragmatic consequences, and as greatly downgrading human interests. But consider, is not a re-balancing of emphasis much more towards animal interests exactly what one might expect that the animals themselves would want communicated to us through their human proxies?

9.3 A Relationship Perspective Addresses Inter-Species Tensions

9.3.1 Seeking reciprocity will enhance commitment to animal care

In an attempt to moderate our tendency to use animals efficiently at the expense of their quality of life, fostering a relationship perspective is recommended. Acknowledging our connection to animals as a social relationship causes an immediate change in perspective which is arguably as dramatic as the shift from examining animals behaviourally from the outside to trying to appreciate their inner experience of subjective states. This is because relationships, as we intuitively understand them, are formed because both parties benefit. Such reciprocal relationships are less stressful to humans (Wolfe, 1985) to the extent that the animal is not as stressed, and this itself increases the pressure on human caretakers to further reduce any stress on the animals. When stress is unavoidable, the relationship requires acknowledgement of this impediment, constant scrutiny to reassess justification and application of every possible safeguard.

In the absence of positive human–animal relationships, there will tend to be negative interactions where humans are stressed and animals are anxious or fearful (e.g. Rushen *et al.*, 1999). Previous attempts to avoid relationships by objectifying animals have not been entirely successful (Arluke, 1992), except to the extent that some beneficiaries of animal use have managed to avoid contact with conscious animals altogether by assigning those duties to other groups, for example researchers/technicians, who must still deal with these issues.

It remains unavoidably apparent, however, that in many cases our use of animals is largely that of exploitation where animals do not experience an actual or perceived benefit. But in acknowledging this fact, and its ethical implications, we must accept some responsibilities. One of these is to consider that those who benefit most directly from such exploitative animal use may not be best placed to judge its necessity. This does not mean, as is claimed by some, that 'Researchers... refuse to address the serious ethical problems of torturing sentient creatures for research purposes. On top of that, over-reliance on animal experimentation has historically hindered scientific advancement' (from The Truth about Vivisection website, www.vivisectioninfo.org). Nor is it true that animal-based researchers, for instance, are driven by a callous desire to complete an experiment no matter what the harm to the animals. Although it is the case that such research does provide personal benefits to those who carry it out by allowing them to satisfy their curiosity or to develop a new theory, the primary justification for the research is invariably, and genuinely, in terms of much wider benefits (Mellor, 1998). However, it is important to ensure that additional non-specialist perspectives are brought to bear on assessments of animal uses that cause harm.

A need for some degree of impartiality in this area is acknowledged. For example, the membership of institutional committees that oversee the use of animals in research, teaching and testing includes independent members from the wider community. Their role is to act as watchdogs on behalf of the animals (e.g. Mellor and Battye, 2000). This principle is further reflected in Ben Mepham's decision-making structure, 'the ethical matrix', in which the views of various stakeholders are spelled out and the final judgement is to be made by an individual who is, as much as possible, blind to their own identity as a member of any of these groups (Mepham, 2000). However, such complete impartiality is not likely because members of the public benefit from most animal use to varying degrees, just as their bonds to the animals involved are felt to varying degrees.

We are often told that uninvolved groups should not make decisions, for example the increasingly urbanized population dictating changes such as the end of fox-hunting in the UK. Yet, this lack of involvement may actually be an asset in ethical decisions relating to other species. Nevertheless, there remains the difficulty that the most involved groups are also those with the greatest level of relevant knowledge. Communication between such groups, especially in helping the general public to understand what the needs of animals are, could be mediated by those animal welfare scientists who can inject a degree of shared, impartial information, without prejudging the final decision (e.g. Mellor and Bayvel, 2008).

9.3.2 Acknowledging and justifying necessary exploitation is challenging

Two widely agreed goals are first, that animals should be given the best life possible within the constraints of their use, and second (which is more implicit), that the benefits of any use should justify the sacrifice made by the animal. Acknowledging the sentience and value of animal life puts appropriate pressure on us to ensure that the purposes of work we do justify the harm (e.g. Mellor, 1998). Attempts to distance ourselves from the animal and minimize its worth may help us to avoid some of our own negative emotional responses to animal exploitation. But it is precisely these negative feelings that motivate us to refine and improve the value, the ethical 'goodness', of the outcomes of our work. There is no easy escape from this ethical responsibility, but realizing that rats are much more like researchers than they are like glass beakers makes our life and choices more emotionally and ethically explicit, and appropriately so, as any discomfort we feel is a necessary part of any non-reciprocal exploitation we choose, no matter how justifiably, to carry out. We have many avenues for remembering and honoring the non-consensual contributions of animals that we deem are necessary (Iliff, 2002).

Therefore, considerations such as this pressurize us to make every relationship with an animal into one of mutual benefit, and this is potentially possible in a wide range of situations. For instance, most people would accept that an owner/pet (guardian/animal) relationship is intended to be mutually beneficial. Many working animals such as sheep dogs show every sign of enjoyment of their way of life and relationship with humans. Equally, non-invasive research may be modelled more upon the owner/pet dynamic than is currently the norm. Advances in enrichment of environments, and retirement of laboratory animals to foster homes mean that some animals in the laboratory gain a net benefit from their use in science, and many more potentially could. Their use in no way requires that their quality of life be as poor as it often currently is.

In considering animals that we exploit, we need some kind of theoretical framework and body of knowledge to draw upon. Currently, most people have very limited ways to conceptualize animals in relationships and so mutual relationships tend to be tagged as 'pet'-like (e.g. Herzog, 2002). However, there are models for respecting exploited animals that are derived from our more agrarian past; that is, from the period prior to our ability to use animals primarily through technological coercion and manipulation. Yet, this body of knowledge is not only largely informal it is fading from collective memory. This includes the role of the farmer as protector of livestock (Serpell, 1999), a role that if acknowledged and synchronized with animal welfare goals makes farmers a very receptive audience. Similar frameworks could be more widely employed by animal caregivers in other arenas such as the laboratory.

In modern agriculture, a smaller proportion of people have direct experience with livestock, and of these many have worked all their lives in intensive, highly engineered systems where the animal has limited opportunities to withdraw its cooperation. Such low levels of experience with (frequently inconvenient) animal behaviour has greatly weakened the natural formation of relationships, and this has been exacerbated by the increased scale of many farms from a few hundred animals to many thousands. Meanwhile in other areas, such as biomedical research, the pre-modern period of husbandry was so brief and localized that only a negligible number of researchers has ever collected rats from the wild or raised them in random breeding colonies kept in large, rubbish-filled rooms. We need to braid together modern sciences and an intuitive understanding of natural history to keep animals under the best conditions possible consistent with their use.

In acknowledging domesticated animals as a subjugated group we take on the responsibility to provide for them. Only in doing so with immaculate skill can we provide an ethically sound basis for suggesting that the exploitation of one sentient being by another may be ethically justified. Currently, some positions in favour of animal exploitation appear to imply a *carte blanche* where any and all uses are allowed that are not sadistically motivated. Although equal obligations properly apply to all animal-based disciplines, animal welfare science perhaps has an additional obligation to provide leadership by always highlighting the requirement to maintain a balance between the need for animal use and the standard of care.

Indeed, an animal welfare position is consistent with recommending the banning of some uses that are of trivial human benefit and a gross imposition on the animals. It is on this basis that some practices such as *foie gras* production, fur-farming and white-veal production are under pressure. Moreover, being in favour of humane animal use is consistent with objecting to the trivialization of animal sacrifices in practices such as drinking goldfish in martinis or using whole chickens or turkeys as bowling balls and cannon balls.

Every animal welfare scientist espouses orientations located somewhere on the continuum between animal advocate and industry advocate. It is not realistic to expect that any one person could obtain some kind of perfect neutrality. What is crucial, however, is that the field as a whole be demonstrably not aligned with either camp, but in a position somewhere between the two, thereby helping to ensure that what the animal-based industries broadly consider to be necessary are conducted in a way that produces the least possible detriment to the animals involved.

9.3.3 Wider perspectives will enhance understanding and ongoing negotiations

A major preoccupation of scientific communities is to change behaviour through discovering and communicating accurate information. But it is not sufficient to merely understand the state of the animal, even if this is expanded to include an understanding of animals' motivations and other internal experiences expressed through behaviour. In many cases, we already have access to sufficient information to provide better conditions for the animal. What then is the obstacle? There are many answers to this question but a great many of them relate to differences between human social cultures; for instance, those concerned with animal welfare, animal users and animal welfare scientists themselves.

Scientists are repeatedly referred to by commentators as 'ethically inarticulate' (Arluke, 1992) or 'ethically naïve' (Mellor, 1998). There is a widespread failure by many researchers to fully appreciate the context within which they do their work. This also extends to understanding the perspectives and beliefs of other groups whose cooperation is necessary for animal care to improve. The answer is not necessarily to require that researchers with a reductionist scientific focus should force themselves to learn the canon of ethics and philosophy; rather, they should seek out and welcome practitioners with different styles, and develop a critical awareness of their disciplines' roles in our society, potentially through the lens of a sociological perspective tempered by ethics (Mellor, 1998).

As scientists we are trained not only to tolerate but also embrace doubt, in that no hypothesis is ever considered absolutely proven, only supported by the current evidence. It is argued here that within animal welfare science ethical doubt about whether or not our use of animals is optimal, appropriate or necessary at all must now be embraced. Retaining such doubt is necessary because not only is our understanding of animal needs imperfect and under development, but also the human need and desire to exploit certain animals is continuing to evolve. Moreover, we must accept that when we use animals in ways that cause them to suffer, we, as their caretakers, will experience negative consequences such as stress and grief (Anonymous, 2001b). In accepting this, we make even exploitive human–animal bonds part of a true relationship, but only to the extent that our emotional well-being is detrimentally affected together with the welfare of the animal, and the extent to which the exploitation is justified by goals we fairly judge to be worth this 'ethical price'.

Part 5
Thinking Outside the Box

Integrated Perspectives

Sleep, Developmental Stage and Animal Welfare

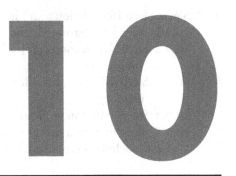

10.1 Introduction

Illustrated here are the benefits of 'thinking outside the box' of the mainstream animal behaviour, welfare and veterinary science disciplines; that is, of keeping an open mind in a scientific discipline sense. It will be shown how searching across disciplines and integrating the knowledge revealed has yielded strikingly fresh insights which have expanded our understanding of factors that can affect animal welfare, in this case sleep.

Insights into the impact of brain development and sleep states before and after birth on animal welfare were derived almost entirely from biomedical literature directed towards improving the clinical management of human fetuses, the birth process and newborn infants, not animal welfare. Likewise, publications on the physiology, psychobiology and pathology of sleep, directed mainly at the better management of human sleep disorders or merely at understanding the fundamentals of sleep and sleep mechanisms, were major sources for the present discussion of sleep and welfare in mature animals, although in this case some animal behaviour and welfare literature was also helpful.

Sleep is a daily experience for each of us. We witness it in ourselves and in animals. We are aware of the compelling drive to sleep when we are tired, of the refreshing benefits of sleeping well, and of irritability, fatigue and other negative feelings when we do not. And, from our knowledge of their behaviour, we assume that sleep is equally important for most livestock, pets and other warm-blooded animals. Yet, with some notable exceptions (e.g. Ruckebusch, 1974; Gallard et al., 1993; Gregory, 1998; Hanninen, 2007), possible roles of sleep in maintaining or restoring animal welfare, or monitoring it, have not received much attention.

As shall be seen, sleep can affect animal welfare directly because, during it, conscious sensory perception is absent or very markedly reduced. This is relevant to young as they develop from immature to mature life stages, and also to adults when challenged by disease states that may be accompanied by sleep. Sleep also has restorative or other beneficial functions in healthy animals and can therefore help to maintain good welfare. In contrast, sleep deprivation leading to fatigue or exhaustion and to increased susceptibility to infections or greater sensitivity to pain may adversely affect welfare. These features of sleep will be examined here, but first some general attributes of sleep will be enumerated.

10.2 General Attributes of Sleep

10.2.1 Sleep is observable in all vertebrates and has particular behavioural attributes

All vertebrates studied to date exhibit sleep or sleep-like behaviour (Meddis, 1975; Karmanova, 1982; Lima *et al.*, 2005), and invertebrates, including crustaceans, molluscs and insects, are also said to exhibit sleep-like behaviour (Meddis, 1975; Lima *et al.*, 2005). Such a wide distribution in the animal kingdom suggests that sleep, or similar behaviours, may have a long evolutionary history. Evidently, therefore, sleep occurs in most species whose welfare may be compromised to an extent that would cause us concern; that is, vertebrates, especially mammals and birds.

Sleep is identified by several general behavioural attributes (Meddis, 1975; Lima *et al.*, 2005). Sleep often occurs at *species-specific sites* and/or with the animal in *species-specific postures*. For instance, animals may sleep in dens, burrows, tall grass or trees, in ground or elevated natural structures or nests, and they may sleep while lying down, standing, perching, swimming or flying. Sleep usually also has a *circadian pattern*, occurring during particular phases of the daily light/dark cycle. A key feature is *inactivity* or *behavioural quiescence*, which may be prolonged, but a sleeping bout may be punctuated by periods of arousal or wakefulness accompanied by grooming and exploration of the sleep site. Typically, during sleep there is an *increased stimulus threshold* for arousal to an alert state, yet sleep is also *rapidly reversible* to conscious wakefulness once arousal has occurred. Finally, *sleep deprivation* elicits a compensatory increase in subsequent sleep, to repay the so-called sleep debt (see below).

The sleep/wake pattern has two main forms in mammals and birds (Lima *et al.*, 2005): *monophasic sleepers*, which tend to sleep during one portion of the day and include human beings and most other primates, and *polyphasic sleepers*, which sleep in several bouts at any time of the day and include many rodents and other small mammals. In addition, some other mammals, such as ungulates, do not fall into one category or the other. Although most birds seem to be monophasic sleepers, waterfowl and shorebirds may be polyphasic. Overall, *daily sleep duration* also varies across species (Meddis, 1975; Siegel, 2005), such that, in general, total hours of sleep are longest in carnivores, intermediate in omnivores, and shortest in herbivores. Sleep duration ranges from 18 to 20 h a day in animals such as the armadillo, bat and North American opossum, through 8–12 h in the cat, dog and pig to 3–5 h in the deer, goat, sheep, horse, giraffe and elephant.

10.2.2 Brain electrical activity has distinctive characteristics during sleep

Sleep is physiologically distinct from conscious wakefulness (Lima *et al.*, 2005; Siegel, 2005). The principal difference relates to the electroencephalogram (EEG). During behavioural signs of sleep, mammals and birds exhibit two basic EEG patterns which differ from the usually low-amplitude high-frequency waves present during conscious wakefulness. The first of these sleep states, non-rapid-eye-movement (non-REM) sleep, also called quiet sleep or slow-wave sleep, is characterized by high-amplitude low-frequency EEG waves and may range from light to deep sleep. The second state is REM sleep, which is also called active sleep or paradoxical sleep. Although the EEG is distinct during REM sleep, it is rather similar to that of alert, awake animals. However, a generalized loss of muscle tone and frequent small muscle twitches, and the rapid eye movements that give it its name, distinguish REM sleep from conscious wakefulness. Non-REM and REM sleep apparently occur in most of the mammals and birds examined to date (Lima *et al.*, 2005; Siegel, 2005).

Sleep appears to be organized into *sleep cycles*, such that non-REM and REM sleep epochs alternate during a given sleep period (Meddis, 1975; Siegel, 2005). During prolonged sleep, deep non-REM sleep usually dominates initially, and REM and lighter non-REM sleep become more prominent later (Lima *et al.*, 2005). The average duration of sleep cycles (non-REM sleep through REM sleep to waking) is strongly correlated with body weight, being short in small animals, for example 8 min in the short-tailed shrew, and long in large ones, for example 1.8 h in the Asiatic elephant (Siegel, 2005).

The vast majority of mammals engage in *bihemispheric sleep*, where both cerebral hemispheres simultaneously exhibit similar non-REM or REM EEG patterns during sleep (Rattenborg *et al.*, 2000; Lima *et al.*, 2005; Siegel, 2005). However, aquatic mammals (cetaceans, eared seals and manatees) and a wide range of bird species can sleep *unihemispherically*; that is, one cerebral hemisphere exhibits non-REM sleep EEG patterns (not REM patterns) and the other wakeful EEG patterns (Rattenborg *et al.*, 2000). In other words, one cerebral hemisphere is asleep, while the other is awake. Although unequivocal states of unihemispheric sleep and conscious wakefulness do occur, intermediate levels of both are also likely. Interestingly, the eye on the side opposite to the sleeping hemisphere is closed and the other eye is open and scanning the environment. Such unihemispheric sleep allows surfacing to breathe in aquatic mammals, and in birds it allows predator detection and possibly migratory or other extended flights (Rattenborg *et al.*, 2000). Finally, birds that engage in unihemispheric sleep also exhibit bihemispheric sleep, with the balance favouring the unihemispheric mode when perceived threats from predators at the sleeping site are high, and bihemispheric sleep when they are not (Rattenborg *et al.*, 2000).

It is worth noting in passing that *hibernation* (that is, prolonged torpor lasting days or weeks) and *shallow daily torpor* are sleep-like states that involve decreases in body and brain temperature to as low as −3 and +12°C, respectively (Deboer and Tobler, 1994). These states are entered via non-REM sleep and although the amplitude of EEG activity decreases during them some non-REM-like activity remains even at the lowest temperatures. These changes in the EEG are considered to reflect the well-known effects of tissue temperature on metabolic rate whereby a 10°C decline in body temperature reduces the rate of chemical processes by a factor of two to three (Deboer, 1998). The question of whether or not hibernation and torpor represent forms of beneficial restorative sleep or states that incur a sleep debt (see below) has yet to be resolved (Heller and Ruby, 2004). Animals are aroused regularly from hibernation and torpor despite the high energy cost of such arousals (Deboer and Tobler, 1994), yet both states are considered to minimize energy demands when environmental nutrient availability is low on a seasonal or daily basis (Kortner and Geiser, 2000). Variants of these states are observed in a range of animals, including some bears, rodents and marsupials, and appear to be appropriate adaptations to their respective ecological niches.

10.2.3 The unconsciousness of sleep, unconscious wakefulness and conscious wakefulness are distinct physiological states

The behavioural and physiological differences between sleep and conscious wakefulness (noted above) show that sleep consists of states of reversible unconsciousness. Chief among these differences are the following: the sleep-specific higher arousal thresholds; the general body immobility during sleep; the distinct EEG patterns together with the presence or absence of associated eye movements, muscle twitches and reductions in muscle tone during sleep; and the capacity to be aroused from sleep to alert or conscious wakefulness. In addition, the high-amplitude low-frequency EEG patterns seen during deep non-REM sleep are also evident in other states of global unconsciousness including general anaesthesia and coma (Baars, 2001; Tung and Mendelson, 2004). However, there is an important caveat; global unconsciousness will occur only if sleep is bihemispheric, because, as we have seen, during unihemispheric sleep one hemisphere remains sufficiently awake to respond to environmental stimuli (Rattenborg et al., 2000).

The unconsciousness of bihemispheric sleep is therefore well established. However, there is potential for confusion regarding the terms 'wakefulness' and 'consciousness', because they are sometimes used as synonyms by sleep researchers. However, there are in fact two distinct physiological states of wakefulness, one is unconscious and the other conscious (Mellor et al., 2005). The distinction depends critically on the extent of engagement of the cerebral cortex. Thus, unconscious wakefulness involves brainstem and thalamic activity, without full cerebral cortical engagement. In contrast, for conscious wakefulness − consciousness − to occur, all incoming information from the body and external environment must be available to all parts of the cerebral cortex at the same time. Thus, it is possible to be awake and not conscious, for example in sleep-walking and sleep-talking, and to be consciously awake, but it is not possible to be asleep and conscious. In the present discussion, therefore, phrases such as conscious wakefulness exclude unconscious wakefulness, and the words wakefulness or awake include both unconscious and conscious forms.

10.3.1 The major pre-conditions of suffering and good welfare are sentience and consciousness

Having considered some general attributes of sleep, wakefulness and consciousness, principally in adult mammals and birds, the possible impacts of the *unconsciousness of sleep* on the welfare of young during their neurobiological development from immature to more mature life stages will now be evaluated.

Let us recall that suffering is the antithesis of good welfare (Chapters 1 and 5). Therefore, in order to suffer (to have poor welfare), and indeed to experience good welfare, an animal must be both sentient and conscious.

10.3.1.1 The animal must be sentient

The nervous system must exhibit sufficient functional sophistication to transduce sensory inputs into positive, neutral or negative sensations or experiences and, with particular regard to unpleasant sensations, the experiences must be of sufficient negative intensity to cause suffering. The capacity for sentience is thought to depend first on the phylogenetic status of the species (Kirkwood, 2006), and second, in those species that exhibit sentience, on the stage of neurological development during the life cycle of the animal (Mellor and Diesch, 2006, 2007). Phylogenetically, all mammals and birds, and probably all other vertebrates, are considered to demonstrate sentience as adults. Accordingly, the focus here will be the developmental stages when the young attain the capacity for sentience, but will be limited to some mammals and birds.

10.3.1.2 Consciousness is also required

Only when an animal is conscious can it experience impulse barrages in sensory nerves according to the modalities of the associated organs; that is, sight, sound, smell, taste, touch, pain and so on. Sleep, as a form of unconsciousness, eliminates conscious perception of all sensory inputs and, if those inputs are sufficiently noxious, it would eliminate any associated suffering provided that the sleep continued. As shall be seen, this has relevance to the welfare of young that have gained the capacity for sentience before birth or hatching, and to other young in which neurological immaturity at birth may delay the subsequent onset of consciousness or awareness.

10.3.2 Neurological immaturity and sleep prevent suffering in mammalian young during pregnancy

There is strong evidence supporting the view that mammalian young initially are not sentient, as they do not have brain structures that are functionally capable of supporting any form of consciousness. Moreover, there is equally compelling evidence that, subsequently, when the capacity for sentience might have developed, the fetus displays EEG activity and behaviour indicating that it is continuously in sleep-like states of unconsciousness. As these observations have been reviewed in detail elsewhere (Mellor and Gregory, 2003; Mellor et al., 2005; Mellor and Diesch, 2006), they will summarized here, with emphasis initially on young that are neurologically mature at birth, for example bovine calves, fawns, foals, kids and lambs.

After fertilization, neural tissue differentiates and then develops via sparsely connected, rudimentary structures into neural aggregations of increasing size and complexity. Thus, as prenatal young develop, peripheral (body) and central (brain) neural structures appear, interconnect and exhibit progressively more sophisticated functional capabilities. Included in this process is the appearance of the sensory structures required for sight, hearing, taste, smell, touch, pain, proprioception and thermal sensitivity. The effective operation of some or all of these senses at birth depends on the extent of neurological maturity achieved by then (see below) and contributes to the survival of the newborn (Mellor and Gregory, 2003). Clearly, if some or all of the associated sense organs are operational immediately after birth, they should have that capacity before birth, and it appears that they do.

The in utero sensory environment is varied and significant, and in late pregnancy fetal sense organs do respond to stimulation in most of the modalities evident at birth (Bradley and Mistretta, 1975). However, although impulse barrages may be elicited in these sense organs this does not necessarily mean that the fetus perceives the associated inputs as sensations. For that to occur, neural states that support consciousness must be present, and three lines of evidence, taken together, strongly suggest that states of unconsciousness persist in the embryo and then the fetus throughout pregnancy and birth. These are outlined below.

10.3.2.1 EEG evidence

Pre-cortical and cortical structures are initially electrically silent. Sporadic electrical spikes and short epochs of sustained EEG activity then appear. Thereafter, continuous undifferentiated EEG activity develops, and this then differentiates into repetitively cycling non-REM and REM sleep-like patterns. It is noteworthy that a capacity for sentience appears when extensive neural connections are made between the thalamus and the cerebral cortex, connections which are critical for consciousness, and that this occurs at around the same time as REM/non-REM sleep-like EEG patterns become evident in the fetus (Lee et al., 2005; Mellor et al., 2005). During labour and birth the balance between these non-REM and REM patterns increasingly shifts towards the deeper non-REM state. Both in terms of their characteristic EEG features and the associated fetal behaviours – the presence or absence of rapid eye movements, muscle twitches and generalized loss of muscle tone – these fetal states are not distinguishable from the non-REM and REM sleep seen after birth. As none of these manifestations of electrical activity in the cerebral cortex is compatible with consciousness in the embryo or fetus at any stage during pregnancy and birth, unconscious states would appear to be continuously present.

10.3.2.2 In utero *neuroinhibitory factors*
There are at least eight fetal, placental and uterine factors, all with well-established inhibitory effects on the fetal EEG, which could contribute to the maintenance of fetal states of sleep-like unconsciousness during the last half of pregnancy, and, in particular, after the capacity for sentience has emerged.

Adenosine Adenosine is a potent neuroinhibitor and sleep-inducing agent, which is present in high concentrations in the fetus, and its tissue concentrations are inversely correlated with the partial pressures of oxygen in fetal tissues.

Allopregnanolone and pregnanolone These are neuroactive steroids with potent anaesthetic, sedative and analgesic (pain-relieving) effects. They are synthesized from progesterone and cholesterol by the fetal brain and placenta, and act via the fetal γ-aminobutyric acid (GABA) neuroinhibitory system.

Prostaglandin D_2 This is a potent sleep-inducing hormone which is also synthesized by the fetal brain and has neuroinhibitory effects.

Placental peptides One or more placental peptides have demonstrated fetal neuroinhibitory effects.

Warmth, cushioned tactile stimulation and buoyancy These three factors are also demonstrably neuroinhibitory.

These neuroinhibitory factors, and possibly others yet to be discovered (Mellor *et al.*, 2005), provide an inhibitory functional environment for the fetal brain, a functional environment which is unique to prenatal life.

10.3.2.3 Non-arousability by potentially noxious stimulation
In striking contrast to healthy newborn and young animals, the fetus is not arousable from non-REM or REM sleep to conscious wakefulness by potentially noxious interventions such as induced hypercapnia (high carbon dioxide), sounds loud enough to cause intense auditory pain and surgery-induced tissue damage. This non-responsiveness is a further indication of the unique inhibitory functional environment of the fetal brain and also suggests that expulsion from the uterus at birth would lead to a marked reduction in overall neuroinhibitory influences on the brain.

  In conclusion, it follows that the welfare of prenatal young is protected initially by an absence of sentience, reflecting neurological immaturity. Once a capacity for sentience does develop in young that will be neurologically mature at birth, welfare is protected by the presence of continuous states of sleep-like unconsciousness that are maintained by a range of well-demonstrated *in utero* neuroinhibitory factors and by an associated non-arousability of the fetus in response to potentially noxious stimulation. These observations have generally reassuring implications for safeguarding welfare while potentially noxious experimental, surgical or clinical procedures are being conducted on the fetus (see Mellor and Gregory, 2003).

10.3.3 Suffering is also prevented during labour and birth

There are two ways fetal suffering is prevented during labour and the expulsion phase of the birth process. The first is that the fetal unconsciousness that has persisted during the last half of pregnancy continues, but with the additional advantage (as noted above) that as labour progresses the balance between non-REM and REM EEG patterns increasingly shifts towards the deeper non-REM state of sleep-like unconsciousness.

The second relates to the complete inability of the fetus to increase its utero-placental oxygen supply from the mother, and to the fact that oxygen supply usually decreases transiently during the uterine contractions of labour (Mellor and Diesch, 2006, 2007). The fetal brain is vulnerable to the deleterious effects of the marked or protracted oxygen shortages which may occur during labour. To avoid brain damage, therefore, the fetus must be able to respond appropriately within its already strictly limited oxygen supply to additional transient or protracted reductions in that supply. This is achieved in part by minimizing muscular activity and the associated increases in oxygen consumption via an explicit maintenance of a physically quiescent state in the fetus throughout labour (Berger et al., 1986; Fraser and Broom, 1990; Hasan and Rigaux, 1991), but this merely decreases background oxygen consumption. However, a potent, rapid-onset neurosuppressive mechanism is also available to the fetus. Thus, if oxygen supply is profoundly reduced or ceases, as may occur with partial or complete occlusion of the umbilical cord between the fetus and the uterine wall during labour contractions, the fetal EEG is reduced to a flat-line (isoelectric) trace within 60–90 s, for example in fetal lambs (Mallard et al., 1992; Bennet et al., 1999; Hunter et al., 2003). This protective mechanism involves adenosine-induced shutdown of electrical activity in the cerebral cortex, which decreases its oxygen consumption and minimizes neural damage if the oxygen shortage is protracted. This suppression is also reversible without harm to cerebral function provided that oxygen supply is reinstated within about 5–6 min. It is worth noting that such neurosuppression may also occur in the newborn after the umbilical cord has been severed and before the onset of breathing reinstates its oxygen supply, if the time taken to start breathing is protracted (Mellor and Diesch, 2006; see below).

It may be concluded that during labour and birth the already unconscious fetus enters deeper states of unconsciousness and becomes physically more quiescent. Moreover, when it is exposed to marked oxygen shortages, it can rapidly and reversibly shut down its cerebrocortical functions. Under these circumstances the fetus could not experience breathlessness due to oxygen shortages, or pain and distress due to compression and tissue injury caused by labour contractions and passage through the birth canal. Nor could it experience any other sensations.

These physiological observations, especially the rapid appearance of a flat-line EEG trace when oxygen supply to the fetus is interrupted, have welcome implications for the management of mature livestock fetuses during slaughter of their pregnant dams, for instance, during the collection of fetal calf serum, and for the humane conduct of fetotomy – dismembering jammed fetuses to resolve intractable labour (Mellor and Gregory, 2003) – as well as for ovariohysterectomy (spay) operations on pregnant companion animals. Thus, provided precautions are taken to ensure that fetal oxygen supply is never reinstated after it has been interrupted such fetuses cannot suffer before they die.

10.3.4 Neurological maturity and the onset of consciousness determine when mammalian young can suffer after birth

The onset of conscious wakefulness, or awareness, after birth depends on the withdrawal of neuroinhibitory factors and increasing involvement of neuroactivators, with these factors operating against a background of the functional maturity of the brain at birth. The mechanisms anticipated to operate in neurologically mature newborns have been detailed elsewhere (Mellor and Gregory, 2003; Mellor *et al.*, 2005; Mellor and Diesch, 2006) and will be summarized below. In addition, the possible impact of various degrees of neurological immaturity at birth on the first appearance of conscious wakefulness after birth will be considered.

10.3.4.1 Neurologically mature young

A delay in the onset of breathing after severance of the umbilical cord will exacerbate any persistent effects of transient oxygen shortages that have occurred during labour, and will lead to a protective adenosine-induced shutdown of EEG activity. However, the successful onset of breathing, stimulated by brainstem reflexes which are safeguarded even during protracted oxygen shortages, will usually restore EEG activity, because re-oxygenating cerebral tissues rapidly reduces adenosine production and its neuroinhibitory effects. Moreover, as breathing becomes well established, tissue oxygenation rises to well above the maximum levels ever achieved before birth, and this will lead to further reductions in adenosine neuroinhibition. It is postulated that this is critical to 'permit' the actions of several neuroactivating factors which have well-demonstrated excitatory effects on the brain (Mellor and Diesch, 2006). These include 17β-oestradiol, which is present in high concentrations during labour and immediately after birth, and noradrenaline, which is released within the brain in response to labour-induced physical compression, pain-receptor input and oxygen shortage. Other neuroactivating factors which come into play after birth include cold, experience of hard surfaces and gravity, maternal grooming, and changes in auditory and visual stimulation. Finally, loss of the placenta at birth contributes to a reduction in neuroinhibition by removing a major source of adenosine, allopregnanolone and pregnanolone (and/or their precursors), and the placental peptide neuroinhibitor(s).

The usual outcome for neurologically mature newborns, including calves, fawns, kids, lambs and foals, is a relatively rapid onset of consciousness after birth (Kilgour and Dalton, 1984; Fraser and Broom, 1990), which nevertheless takes some minutes to occur (Mellor and Gregory, 2003; Mellor and Stafford, 2004; Figures 10.1, 10.2 and 10.3). Thus, there are no behavioural signs of consciousness while the newborn lies immobile on the ground immediately after birth. Nor is consciousness evident when the newborn first lifts and/or shakes its head and gasps as a prelude to the onset of breathing. Even soon after rhythmic breathing has been established, when the newborn lies in sternal recumbency holding its head up, the presence of unconscious wakefulness and not consciousness seems more likely. Vocalization

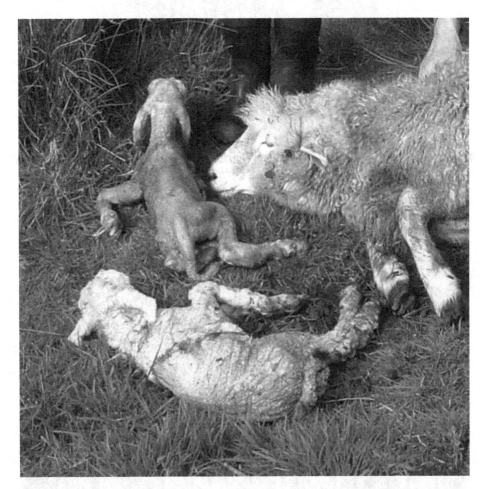

Figure 10.1 Twin lambs immediately after the birth of the second lamb. The lamb born first, several minutes before, is lying normally and holding its head up, while the second lamb is lying on its side and just beginning to lift its head (©2009, M. Oliver, reproduced with permission).

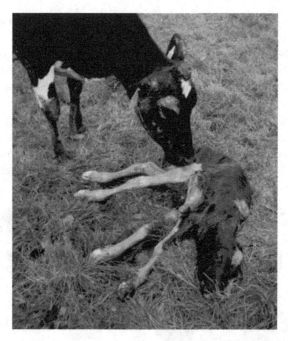

Figure 10.2 A calf lying flat on the ground immediately after birth, before it starts to breathe (©2009, T.J. Diesch, reproduced with permission).

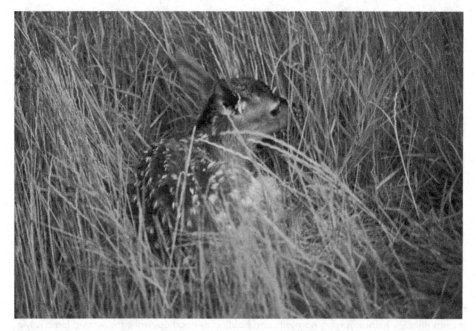

Figure 10.3 A conscious red deer fawn lying in grass within 2 h of birth (©2009, M.W. Fisher, reproduced with permission).

may occur at this stage. The subsequent responsiveness of the newborn to maternal attention and its initial fruitless attempts to stand followed by successful standing and teat-seeking activity may all be signs of continuing unconscious wakefulness or could represent very early signs of conscious wakefulness. A progression from these states towards alert consciousness, assessed behaviourally, becomes apparent only after this.

More precise estimates of the time when *un*consciousness first disappears after birth could be obtained from EEG data which, unfortunately, are not apparently available. Nevertheless, the analysis above suggests that the newborn may progress from initial EEG shutdown and/or sleep-like unconsciousness through unconscious wakefulness and then to conscious wakefulness. It also seems likely that any conscious wakefulness experienced by the newborn within minutes of birth would be more muted than the alert consciousness it exhibits when fully awake at, for instance, 12–24 h after birth. Thus, an almost immediate switch to alert consciousness is not likely. A gradual shift may in part be due to a postnatal continuation of the cerebral synthesis of two neuroactive steroids, allopregnanolone and pregnanolone, which, as noted above, probably contribute to maintaining the sleep-like EEG states in the fetus by virtue of their well-demonstrated anaesthetic and sedative actions (Mellor *et al.*, 2005). Such actions in the newborn are likely to be highest immediately after birth, and wane in parallel with the circulating concentrations of allopregnanolone, which are known to decrease during the first 1–3 days after birth in lambs (Mellor and Diesch, 2006).

It is against this background that we need to assess the potential for neurologically mature newborns to suffer. Newborns that never achieve consciousness, for instance those that never breathe successfully, would die without suffering. Gasping, kicking and head lifting in such newborns are therefore not a cause for welfare concern. Nor is welfare of concern before consciousness appears in those newborns that do breathe successfully. Even during the transitional phase of muted consciousness we might anticipate that the newborn is afforded some protections against suffering, but this has yet to be investigated rigorously. However, once conscious wakefulness becomes established there is likely to be much greater potential for suffering to occur if sensory inputs are sufficiently noxious. Nevertheless, some protective factors may still be present. For instance, the persistent, though waning, cerebral synthesis of allopregnanolone and pregnanolone during the first few days after birth may, through their analgesic actions, reduce the experience of pain associated with birth-induced injuries. Such analgesia may also contribute to the lower noxious sensory input caused by castration in lambs within 1–3 days of birth compared to that in older lambs (Johnson *et al.*, 2009). The sedative actions of these neuroinhibitory steroids may contribute to the relative inactivity of the young that is regularly seen in the absence of threatening stimuli during the first day after birth. Such relative inactivity facilitates maternal grooming and helps to establish a strong mother–young bond with its associated protective benefits. Finally, hypothermia – a lower than normal body temperature – is a common state in newborn ungulates born in temperate climates, and, when present, is anticipated to dull consciousness and thereby to alleviate noxious experiences (Mellor and Stafford, 2004).

10.3.4.2 Neurologically immature young

The development of brain functionality appears to follow a broadly similar path in mammalian young whatever their neurological maturity at birth, and this is reflected in the EEG (Ellingson and Rose, 1970). Thus, an initial electrical silence in the precortical and cortical structures is first punctuated by intermittent spikes and then short epochs of more sustained activity. Continuous undifferentiated EEG activity then becomes established and this later differentiates into repetitively cycling non-REM and REM sleep-like patterns. Finally, the EEG of conscious wakefulness is added once the young reach the age when daily sleep/wake cycles appear.

The stage when birth occurs during this developmental path depends on the species and obviously, therefore, determines the neurological maturity of the young at birth (Table 10.1). As we have seen, the most neurologically mature newborns pass through all but the last of these developmental stages before birth. At the other extreme, newborn marsupial joeys are neurologically exceptionally imma-ture, and most development occurs postnatally while they are in their mother's pouch (Tyndale-Biscoe and Janssens, 1988). In the tammar wallaby, for example, after a 28–32-day pregnancy, the joey occupies the pouch for about 250 days. Its EEG evidently remains electrically silent until about 100–120 days of in-pouch age and becomes continuous by about 150–160 days, and behavioural signs of conscious wakefulness are apparent by about 160–180 days (Tyndale-Biscoe and Janssens, 1988; Diesch et al., 2008; Figure 10.4). Newborn rat pups are also neurologically immature, but markedly less so than newborn joeys. Their EEG has been described as isoelectric or of very low voltage at birth, and intermittent or continuous but undifferentiated between birth and 5–8 days after birth; REM/non-REM differentiation occurs between days 12 and 18, and EEG evidence for conscious wakefulness is apparent no earlier than this (Ellingson and Rose, 1970; Snead and Stephens, 1983; Diesch et al., 2009). A similar EEG status at birth and similar subsequent patterns of development have also been reported in the young of the cat (Figure 10.5), dog, mouse and rabbit, although the precise timing differs in each case (Ellingson and Rose 1970).

In view of the requirement for sentience and conscious wakefulness to be present before sensory inputs can be experienced as positive, neutral or negative (see above), young that are neurologically immature at birth presumably cannot suffer when exposed to potentially noxious stimulation at the postnatal ages when the EEG indicates the absence of conscious wakefulness. If it is conserva-tively assumed that conscious wakefulness cannot occur postnatally any earlier than the age when REM/non-REM differentiation is first evident – when critical corticothalamic connections are made (see above) – the welfare of neurologically immature young appears to be protected after birth for about the first 4 days in

Table 10.1 EEG features indicating different levels of neurological maturity in some mammalian young at birth and avian young at hatching.

	Stage of neurological development		
EEG features	**Exceptionally immature**	**Immature**	**Mature**
	Electrical silence → Spikes–short epochs →	Continuous →	REM/non-REM sleep → Sleep/wake cycles
Mammalian young	←	↑ ↑ ↑	←
	Marsupial joey	Kitten	Calf
		Puppy	Fawn
		Mouse pup	Foal
		Rat pup	Kid
		Rabbit kit	Lamb
			Piglet
			Guinea pig pup
Avian young	←		←
	Pigeon		Domestic chicken

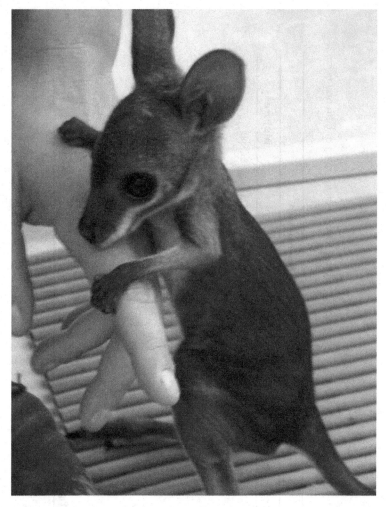

Figure 10.4 A tammar wallaby joey at 170–190 days of in-pouch age (©2009, T.J. Diesch, reproduced with permission).

the rabbit, 7 days in the cat, 10 days in the rat and mouse and, possibly depending on the breed, for 4–14 days in the dog (see Ellingson and Rose, 1970). Arousal or so-called 'wake' behaviours (largely muscular movements) that may be observed before REM/non-REM differentiation occurs are not a cause for concern because the EEG, when measured, indicates the persistence of unconsciousness. Clearly, this protected period is much longer in the young of marsupial species, being about 150 days in tammar wallaby joeys (see above).

These observations have implications for the acceptability or otherwise of conducting invasive procedures on such newborns without anaesthesia. They suggest,

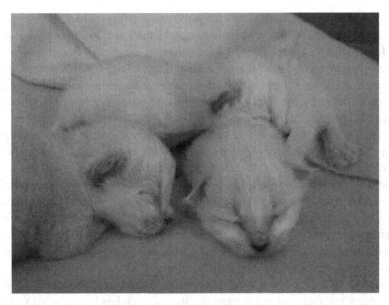

Figure 10.5 Three kittens within 3 days of birth, about 7 days before eye-opening normally occurs (©2009, L. Wilkinson, reproduced with permission).

for instance, that tail docking may not lead to *perceived* pain in puppies aged less than 4–14 days, depending on the breed, but confirmation of this would require EEG evidence that such puppies are not aroused to conscious wakefulness. Persistent unconsciousness seems likely, however, in view of the conservative cut-off criterion of only conducting such procedures before the onset of REM/non-REM differentiation and the associated step in neurological development.

10.3.5 The pattern and implications of neurological development are somewhat similar in mammalian and avian species

Guided by the insights noted above regarding factors that influence the onset of conscious wakefulness in mammalian young, the possible implications of the parallel development of some neurological features in pre-hatched and hatched domestic chickens have also been evaluated (Mellor and Diesch, 2007), and the key conclusions are recorded here.

Although the process takes about 21 days in the chick and about 21 weeks in the lamb, the general patterns of behavioural, neuroanatomical and neurophysiological development in the chick before hatching and in the lamb before birth are strikingly similar, and, overall, the developmental pattern of the EEG also seems to be similar in both species (Table 10.1). Thus, the chick appears to be insentient for the first 16–17 days of incubation, during which initial EEG silence is later punctuated by spikes or short epochs of more sustained activity, and then continuous undifferentiated sleep-like activity appears. Thereafter, repetitively cycling REM/non-REM patterns become established and are maintained between about day 19 and hatching. Thus, if similar neurobiological foundations operate in the developing avian and mammalian brains, the capacity for sentience may appear in pre-hatched chicks by about day 19. However, as in the neurologically mature fetus, neuroinhibitory mechanisms apparently also operate in pre-hatched chicks, helping to keep them unconscious.

Epipregnanolone, a neuroactive steroid, is synthesized by the avian brain and acts via the GABA inhibitory system, and is anticipated to have anaesthetic and sedative properties in the chick which are similar to those of its mammalian fetal equivalents (allopregnanolone and pregnanolone). Warmth is also neuroinhibitory, as reversal of cold exposure elicits specific behavioural and EEG responses that indicate less arousal in mature chicks near hatching. A dearth of published information prevents assessment of the potential involvement in chicks of the other neuroinhibitory factors that are effective in fetuses (see above). However, there is an additional mechanism, apparently unique to birds, which involves neuro-inhibitory effects of the chick's neck becoming folded as is grows within the egg. Thus, asymmetrical neural input from the folded neck has been shown to promote sleep-like EEG activity and to inhibit arousal responses to otherwise potent arousing stimuli.

This folded-neck inhibition may have an important overriding effect because, unlike the fetus, the chick *in ovo* can, and indeed must, increase its oxygen supply to support the increased muscular activity required for hatching behaviour and escape from the egg. It does this initially by penetrating the air-space membrane (called *internal pipping*) to allow access to the air space within the egg. The chick then starts to breathe that air. This somewhat enhances its oxygen supply, which previously is met entirely via the chorioallantoic membrane and gas exchange across the eggshell. Before the onset of vigorous hatching behaviour, oxygen supply via breathing is enhanced even more when the chick makes a hole in the eggshell (called *external pipping*), thereby allowing it direct access to the higher oxygen content of atmospheric air. Such increases in oxygen supply might be expected to decrease adenosine-induced neuroinhibition in the chick. There is apparently no published information on the chick's adenosine status during hatching, but overriding neuroinhibitory effects of the folded neck could help to maintain sleep-like unconsciousness during hatching. That this is likely is supported by the observation that refolding conscious hatched chicks with extended necks into glass eggs produces sleep-like EEG states and reduced arousal responses. Nevertheless, some vocal–auditory interactions between the mother and chick before and during hatching may suggest that there is some level of pre-hatching consciousness in the chick. While the EEG evidence tends to contradict this, and alternative explanations can be provided, the question of consciousness at this late stage of incubation does merit further investigation (Mellor and Diesch, 2007).

After hatching the chick usually takes at least 2 h, and possibly longer, before it exhibits sustained behavioural and EEG evidence of conscious wakefulness (Mellor and Diesch, 2007). Note, however, that its EEG is relatively mature at hatching. Pigeon chicks, on the other hand (Table 10.1), apparently exhibit EEG silence during the first 3 days, and there is a slow evolution of the EEG to more mature forms between days 6 and 14. This slower developmental pattern has been attributed to greater cerebral cortical immaturity in the hatchling pigeon than in the domestic chick (Ellingson and Rose, 1970). The range of neurological maturity at hatching suggested by these few observations in avian species (also see Rogers, 1995) may therefore parallel that seen in mammalian young at birth (marsupials excluded) (Table 10.1). This appears to merit further investigation.

10.3.6 These fresh insights and their wider implications need to be assessed experimentally

It is important to consider the status of the observations made above. They are fresh insights based on recent integrative syntheses of well-demonstrated, yet not well-known, findings in the scientific literature (Mellor and Gregory, 2003; Mellor *et al.*, 2005; Mellor and Diesch, 2006, 2007), some of which date back 30–40 years. Although the literature provides a compelling case for persistent unconsciousness before birth or hatching, this proposition is nevertheless contrary to views held firmly by many people. In light of this, a major purpose of presenting this alternative view, and the supporting scientific evidence, is to stimulate others to challenge them experimentally. If this view survives such challenges it may then be adopted more widely. Whatever the outcome, the evidence presented already exists in the literature and needs to be assimilated into our understanding of developmental processes in young before and after birth and hatching.

10.3.6.1 Use of pain relief in the fetus

These observations raise questions regarding whether or not, when and how pain relief – anaesthesia and/or analgesia – should be provided when invasive procedures are conducted on young at different stages of their neurological development. In light of a dearth of information on these matters, current pressure to provide pain relief to mammalian fetuses during surgery requires careful consideration, and a cautious approach is recommended to avoid untoward effects of the pain-relieving drugs on the young (Diesch *et al.*, 2008; Mellor *et al.*, 2008a).

10.3.6.2 Impact of maternal death on the fetus

There are also implications related to the impact on fetuses of killing the pregnant dam, and the precautions required when killing newborn or young animals before the ages when they become conscious.

Oxygen supply to the fetus ceases with death of the dam. This usually elicits a burst of fairly vigorous physical activity by the fetus, but as such behavioural responses begin during the early stages of neurological development when the EEG is electrically silent, they are considered to be spinal or lower-brain-centre reflexes, which are perhaps designed to free a compressed umbilical cord and restore oxygen supply (Bennet et al., 1999, 2003). Thus, fetal movement after death of the dam is not a sign of distress or suffering in early fetuses. Nor is it in fetuses later in pregnancy. This conclusion is fully supported for all fetuses, whatever their stage of neurological development at the time of maternal death, by the EEG evidence outlined here which shows that they remain in continuous states of unconsciousness throughout pregnancy. Moreover, in fetuses that are neurologically mature at birth, cessation of oxygen supply during late pregnancy after REM/non-REM differentiation has occurred causes complete suppression of the fetal EEG within 60–90 s; that is, the EEG rapidly becomes electrically silent (Mallard et al., 1992; Watson et al., 2002; Hunter et al., 2003). This means that even after the capacity for sentience has developed in neurologically mature fetuses, the suppressive effects of a cessation of oxygen supply guarantee that the already unconscious fetus rapidly enters a brain state that is totally incompatible with consciousness (Mellor and Gregory, 2003). On the basis of these observations, therefore, it may be concluded that fetal distress and suffering do not occur after maternal death whatever the stage of fetal neurological maturity. There is one caveat for neurologically mature fetuses. When maternal death occurs close to birth, exposed fetuses must be prevented from successfully breathing air because their more mature lungs may enable them to elevate their brain oxygen to levels that are compatible with consciousness (Mellor and Gregory, 2003; Mellor, 2003). Leaving all such fetuses in the uterus until they are dead achieves this objective, although other precautions allow earlier exposure (Mellor, 2003; van der Valk et al., 2004).

These impacts on the fetus are independent of the method used to kill the dam, assuming of course that those methods are humane. Thus, anaesthetic overdose, carbon dioxide or inert-gas inhalation, effective stunning followed by transverse neck-cut exsanguination, a well-executed captive bolt or free-bullet head-shot, and other humane methods applied to the dam would pose no concerns regarding the welfare of the fetus as it dies. This is also true for fetuses during ovariohysterectomy (spay) of the pregnant uterus.

10.3.6.3 Euthanasia of newborn and young animals
Euthanasia of neurologically immature newborn and young animals, which have not yet achieved consciousness, would appear on the face of it to be quite straightforward as they normally cannot experience pain, distress or any other sensations. However, several factors may complicate our response to this. Such young can locate the dam and begin to drink milk soon after birth, and they may exhibit physical and vocal responses to invasive stimuli. For many people such behaviour seems to belie the notion that the young are unconscious. Also, our natural, possibly inbuilt, inclination to care for and protect vulnerable young may inhibit us from killing them even if we can do so without causing pain and distress. One solution is to always employ euthanasia methods that would be acceptable

if used in older conscious animals, methods that ensure progress towards death is smooth and without worrisome behavioural responses. Clearly, that principle also applies to the choice of euthanasia method for young that are neurologically mature at birth.

10.4 Sleep, Sleep Deprivation and the Welfare of Mature Animals

In view of the significant place sleep has in the daily rest/activity cycles of animals and the well-recognized detrimental effects of sleep deprivation or disturbance (Meddis, 1975; Lima *et al.*, 2005; Bonnet, 2005; Siegel, 2005) it is surprising that until recently possible relationships between sleep and animal welfare have not received much attention.

It is logical to assume that several facets of animal welfare would be linked to the functions or *benefits* of sleep. For instance, it is argued that the behavioural immobility of sleep is a major survival stratagem deployed in various ways depending on the animal's ecological niche (Meddis, 1975). Thus, the global unconsciousness of bihemispheric sleep in those animals that display it and the retained capacity for environmental scanning in animals that exhibit unihemispheric sleep are said to reflect the physiological elements that underlie this survival function of sleep (Lima *et al.*, 2005; Siegel, 2005). In animal welfare terms, it follows that, in general, prey animals will benefit by using sleep to avoid predation and the associated pain and distress, and predators benefit by being consciously awake at optimal hunting times, which helps them to avoid starvation and the associated marked hunger. However, the focus here is on the internal or functional benefits of sleep and their welfare consequences for individual animals, not the possible evolutionary significance of sleep.

10.4.1 Sleep has restorative and other beneficial functions

Sleep may be considered to be part of a self-regulatory (homeostatic) response to the physiological cost of conscious wakefulness, a cost that may be expressed in terms of *sleep debt*. In general, the sleep debt builds in proportion to the duration of consciousness (Siegel, 2005), with additive effects from physical or psychological challenges experienced while consciously awake (Smith, 1985), and the debt must be repaid with additional amounts of sleep. Although the physiological basis of sleep debt remains poorly understood, the greater the debt is the greater is the *drive to sleep*, and this is experienced as ranging in intensity from normal sleepiness through fatigue to exhaustion. In animal welfare terms, situations that lead to the experience of fatigue may be, and those that lead to exhaustion would be, matters of concern.

A number of beneficial effects of sleep on brain functionality and metabolic activity have been identified. For instance, brain glycogen stores, depleted during wakefulness, are restored (Benington and Heller, 1995) and anabolic (synthetic) processes accelerate (Shapiro and Flanigan, 1993) during non-REM sleep. More generally within the body, during non-REM sleep overall metabolic rate and body temperature decrease, thereby conserving energy (Shapiro and Flanigan, 1993). There is evidence that REM and/or non-REM sleep contributes to learning and the consolidation of memory (Smith, 1985; Stickgold, 2005), although this has been contested (Vertes, 2004). Also, REM sleep, which predominates during early development, may have a key role in the generation of new nerve cells in the developing brain (Siegel, 2005). Finally, the high proportion of each day newborn and young animals spend asleep, and therefore virtually immobile, also favours partitioning nutrient distribution within the body towards tissue growth as opposed to energetically expensive muscular activity.

10.4.2 Sleep deprivation can lead to profound animal welfare compromise

Sleep deprivation has many forms (Bonnet, 2005). It can be short term or long term, partial or total, or aimed at a particular sleep phase (non-REM or REM). Quite apart from its deleterious effects on mental function, manifested in human beings as irritability, poor concentration, confusion, disorientation and feelings of exhaustion, sleep deprivation has other adverse effects, including disruptions to immune defences, hormonal secretion, energy balance and body temperature control. When sleep deprivation is prolonged, for example for 1 month in rats, these functional disruptions can be severe enough to cause death (Toth, 1995; Bonnet, 2005). Although it is not clear to what extent these effects result from the sleep deprivation itself or the associated activation of stress responses in the sleep-deprived animals (Toth, 1995), the overall outcome is one of severe animal welfare compromise. This extreme case illustrates the possibility that less-severe sleep deprivations may increase the vulnerability of animals to other adverse events, including for instance, exposure to infectious disease agents.

Sleep deprivation in animals may be produced by a range of human interventions; for example small tether stalls for veal calves and stalls for larger sows may prevent them from using their preferred sleeping position. Many settings such as dog shelters are very noisy and may disrupt normal sleeping patterns. Poultry housing may use intermittent or other unnatural patterns of lighting. Transportation is also a major disruptor of sleep largely through movement and vibration. Humans may even disrupt sleep directly such as by using dogs on shift work (Adams and Johnson, 1994) and disturbing wildlife through sound pollution (helicopters, fireworks) or a desire to watch wildlife at their resting and sleeping sites. Many nocturnal laboratory animals (and pets) are routinely disturbed and handled during their sleep period, although, notwithstanding human convenience and health and safety considerations, it is relatively simple to reverse the light cycle of a housing facility. Any decrease in thermal or physical comfort, lack of bedding or proximity of predatory species, such as in an adjoining zoo exhibit, may reduce the quality or quantity of sleep. As sleep deprivation often occurs indirectly and leaves no obvious direct physical damage it may be largely unappreciated as a cause of welfare compromise.

10.4.3 Sleep affects and is affected by defence responses to infectious microorganisms

The impact of sleep on susceptibility to infection with microorganisms, the impact of such infections on sleep, and the potential for sleep to enhance recovery from such infections have been considered in detail elsewhere (Toth, 1995; Gregory, 1998). Briefly, the major conclusions are as follows. First, sleep deprivation appears to reduce the effectiveness of the body's resistance (immune defences) to invading microorganisms, possibly because of the associated stress responses or metabolic disturbances, or both. Conversely, sleep seems to promote disease resistance. Second, infected animals initially exhibit enhanced non-REM sleep concurrently with fever. This sleep enhancement has been linked to some fever-inducing cytokines which are released as part of the immune response to infection and which also appear to have specific sleep-inducing effects. Third, as sleep deprivation during the initial stages of infection can lead to higher mortality or more prolonged morbidity (sickness), sleep appears to facilitate recovery from microbial infections either by promoting immune defences or by aiding recuperation, or both. These beneficial effects are thought to be due to enhanced disease resistance achieved through a sleep-induced reduction in stress which would otherwise impair immune defences, but this has yet to be confirmed. Fourth, the observations above relate more to infections that largely affect non-neural organs and tissues, because qualitatively more diverse sleep abnormalities tend to arise with microorganisms that target neural tissue if they disrupt brain function, for example rabies virus.

It follows that sleep may benefit animal welfare by helping to maintain disease resistance and by facilitating recovery and recuperation from infection. Moreover, while animals are asleep they do not experience unpleasant sensations associated with the infections themselves, nor possible responses to them, including any pain, irritation or distress associated with inflammation of target tissues such as the lungs, digestive organs, genital tract and skin. Conversely, potentially stressful situations which also disrupt sleep, such as long-distance road transport or long-term exposure to uncongenial environmental noise, may predispose animals to infections and their untoward effects. These observations suggest that there would be merit in giving more attention to links between sleep, infection and recovery and their implications for animal welfare.

10.4.4 Sleep–pain interactions can affect animal welfare status

Pain can be a noxious experience with a considerable negative impact on animal welfare status. It is therefore of interest to consider factors that modulate the experience of pain, including sleep. An exploration of relationships between sleep, sleep disturbance or deprivation and pain sensitivity in human beings and animals (Lautenbacher et al., 2006) permits the following general comments to be made.

Pain may disrupt sleep by eliciting arousal and neurological stress responses which are incompatible with undisturbed sleep, and disturbed sleep may itself increase pain sensitivity by decreasing the threshold to pain stimulation. A self-reinforcing situation may therefore arise which may start with disturbed sleep or pain, where these two components either maintain or augment each other. This raises the prospect of two pain-relieving strategies related to sleep enhancement; one is to focus on relieving the pain with analgesics, and the other is to focus on managing the disturbed sleep, for example using sedatives, where both strategies have the purpose of promoting restorative sleep in order to facilitate pain relief in the longer term. There is also the prospect that, in affecting some cerebral mechanisms that are normally involved in sleep, several general anaesthetics may be used temporarily to facilitate the restorative functions of sleep in clinical situations, such as intensive care units, in which significant sleep disturbance is likely (Tung and Mendelson, 2004).

10.4.5 Sleep may be a useful index of animal welfare status

The presence or absence of sleep or conscious wakefulness, together with numerous other behaviours (e.g. Morton and Griffiths, 1985), is regularly used in general or clinical assessments of the health and welfare status. We have already seen that some responses to infections induce sleep and that strongly aversive environments or pain may prevent it. However, changes in the duration, pattern (distribution within the day) and character (non-REM, REM) of sleep may offer opportunities to detect more subtle perturbations, for instance in animals' adaptive responses to less extreme environmental challenges (Ruckebusch, 1975; Smith, 1985; Hanninen, 2007). Although electronic monitoring of the different attributes of sleep (duration, pattern, character) may be accomplished relatively easily in experimental settings, it would be much more difficult in veterinary clinics and completely impractical in the home or field. Nevertheless, experimental demonstrations of changes in sleep attributes and how long it takes for them to stabilize in different configurations or return to the previous one could help identify informative behavioural indices and/ or practical management strategies which could then be used without electronic monitoring. As animals endeavour to maintain their usual sleep period over longer periods, changes in the attributes of sleep may need to be used more subtly to assess chronic conditions, and negative results should be interpreted cautiously. Despite the complexities it would be worthwhile to explore the potential to use changes in the attributes of sleep as additional indices of animals' responses to and recovery from a range of challenging situations.

10.4.6 Concluding remarks concerning sleep

Sleep is an important behaviour for most animal species not only because it occupies a significant part of the day but also because its quality and quantity can be an index of environment suitability and comfort, and disruptions to it have both immediate and long-term effects on overall welfare. Because sleep is an unconscious state for us it may be easy to underestimate the emphasis that should be placed on sleep as one of the major ingredients of a healthy ethogram and an important aspect of a good quality of life. However, sleeplessness should be seen as a fundamental state of suffering equivalent to other discomfort states such as physical exhaustion, thermal discomfort, or hunger, albeit one that is often more difficult to appreciate or diagnose. Direct methods for measuring sleep as a state (as opposed to rest or immobility) and identifying it as a root cause of behavioural and health symptoms should be more widely employed to refine the many practices that have the potential to disrupt normal sleep positions and patterns. Fundamental sleep research also aids our understanding of neurological states that modify an animal's ability to suffer.

The Wider Context of Animal Welfare Science

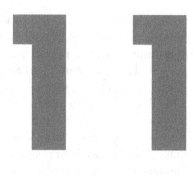

Interest in caring for animals has an exceptionally long history. Even in antiquity it seems that animals and the way people interacted with them were observed by others in order to enhance the capacity of animals to meet human needs. A strictly scientific interest in animal care is more recent. It arose as methods evolved progressively from impressionistic observations into hypothesis-driven and manipulative investigations that included the key elements of quantitation, repeatability, and objective reasoning and critique. The result has been the emergence during the last century of a range of animal-based scientific disciplines, which, as outlined above, underpin and continue to contribute to the more recently emerged discipline of animal welfare science.

Animal welfare science – the discipline concerned with the acquisition and application of the knowledge required to characterize, maintain, restore and promote animal welfare – has had a positive impact to date. Nevertheless, as with all other disciplines, its establishment with dedicated degree courses, textbooks, journals, research departments and specialists, carries with it the risk of creating a form of limiting orthodoxy. This might involve an increase in the fundamental assumptions that are adopted and disseminated, and a narrowing of the range of past and present sources consulted, the colleagues included, the philosophies represented and the techniques employed. It might also involve placing an increasing focus on performing a professional role rather than extending the innovative base of the discipline.

Students, who are usually scientifically naïve, may be particularly vulnerable to the limiting consequences of any tendency among their instructors towards discipline orthodoxy. This is because students initially have an uncritical desire to master the language and reasoning of what is a totally new area of knowledge for them. A counter to this is to show them how present-day thinking is rooted in past ideas in an unbroken sequence that will project into the future, as has been attempted here. The purpose is to illustrate that no ideas are fixed and immutable – all may be reinterpreted, changed markedly or discarded – yet at any one time it is possible to act responsibly within the constraints of what is then current understanding. Indeed, students can be invited to consider themselves as preparing to be participants in and future contributors to the flux of ideas that characterizes their chosen discipline. And the more open the thinking is that contributes to that flux, the more vital and exciting will be the discipline, in this case animal welfare science.

The scientific base of animal welfare science is diverse. It includes animal husbandry, biochemistry, genetics, immunology, nutrition, physiology, pharmacology, plant and soil sciences, veterinary pathology, veterinary clinical sciences and, especially at present, animal behaviour science and cognitive-neural sciences. This discipline diversity provides the comprehensive foundations of our current understanding of the factors that determine the internal experiential state of an animal that represents its welfare, as outlined in this book. Although coping with this diversity may be somewhat daunting for established scientists, let alone students, it is important for them to be aware of and, if possible, to contribute to the free-ranging exploratory originality that is quite often generated at the frontiers where disciplines intersect. It is also important to recognize that the implications of animal welfare extend well beyond the scientific pursuits that help us to better understand and manage it.

Animal welfare is a matter of significant social concern so that in the wider decision-making context, for instance with regard to formulating national policies and codes of practice, it also embraces elements of ethics, philosophy, psychology, sociology, economics, politics and law (Webster, 1994, 2005b; Mellor and Bayvel, 2004; Turner and D'Silva, 2006). Clearly, even the most accomplished of individuals would have exceptional difficulty in managing this diversity in its entirety. One solution is to ensure that all, or most, of the areas required are covered by different experts at institutional, regional or national level, and that an ethos of inclusiveness, open communication and mutual respect is fostered by individuals who have leadership roles in integrating and encouraging constructive participation across the board (Mellor and Battye, 2004; Mellor and Bayvel, 2004, 2008).

Although it is important not to exaggerate the role of animal welfare science in the wider societal context, it is equally important to acknowledge the substantial contribution it continues to make via its multidisciplinary base. It is no accident that animal welfare laws in Australia, Canada, the European Union, New Zealand, the UK and elsewhere emphasize scientific validation as a key factor in determining the minimum welfare standards that are included in codes of practice (e.g. Mellor and Bayvel, 2008; Veissier *et al.*, 2008). Likewise, the global animal welfare guidelines developed and promulgated by the World Organisation for Animal Health (the OIE) on behalf of its 172 member countries and territories similarly highlight scientific validation (Bayvel, 2006; Fraser D, 2008). Scientific literacy, or at least access to clear scientific explanation, is therefore important in the animal welfare arena. There are opportunities for animal welfare scientists to contribute here.

Clear benefits would be obtained if many more animal welfare scientists were to disburse from academia into the realms of national and local government, regional regulatory agencies, primary industries, food manufacturing and distribution companies, funding agencies, animal charities, non-governmental organizations including humane societies and animal rights groups, and other such entities. A small number of influential scientists in a few national or international organizations are not sufficient to provide the required scientific support in every significant area where animals are used. Whenever animal-use decisions are made, animal welfare scientists need to be directly involved, and this should become so routine that their participation is actively solicited.

Such participation would build upon benefits that have already accrued from the establishment of animal welfare science as a discipline. For instance, rigorous scientific perspectives have helped to enhance and legitimize concern for animals within society generally and at the highest levels of key national and international organizations (Bayvel, 2006; Ryan, 2006; Mellor and Bayvel, 2008), so that the discipline has become a major contributor to the transition from grassroots empathetic concern for animals at local level to the beginnings of global change (Turner and D'Silva, 2006; Fraser D, 2008; Rushen, 2008). Although these are significant achievements, the contribution made by animal welfare science should be kept in perspective. The science is an instrument, albeit a very important one, for understanding what animal welfare is and, importantly, how it can be assessed, maintained, compromised and restored. However, value judgements about the acceptability or otherwise of treating animals in particular ways are not primarily scientific; they involve various combinations of ethical, cultural, social, political, legal, economic and other such wider societal considerations, as well as scientific understanding (Mellor and Bayvel, 2004, 2008).

In common with many animal welfare scientists and others, we, the authors of this book, have come to understand that animal welfare problems are problems *for* the animals, but problems often caused by, and which therefore must be solved by, people. It will be important to ensure, however, that human-centred interests represented in the wider societal context do not distract us from the animal-centred focus that will be essential for the solutions devised to genuinely improve the welfare of the animals themselves.

References

Abbott, N.C., White, A.R. and Ernst, E. (1996) Complementary medicine. *Nature* **381**, 361.

Adams, G.J. and Johnson, K.G. (1994) Sleep, work and the effects of shift work in drug detector dogs *Canis familiaris*. *Applied Animal Behaviour Science* **41**, 115–26.

Ader, R. (1965) Effects of early experience and differential housing on behavior and susceptibility to gastric erosions in the rat. *Journal of Comparative Physiology and Psychology* **60**, 233–8.

Aitken, I.D. (ed.) (2007) *Diseases of Sheep*, 4th edn. Blackwell Science, Oxford.

Alroe, H.F., Vaarst, M. and Kristensen, E.S. (2001) Does organic farming face distinctive livestock welfare issues? A conceptual analysis. *Journal of Agricultural and Environmental Ethics* **14**, 275–99.

Anderson, B. (1995) Dendrites and cognition: a negative pilot study in the rat. *Intelligence* **20**, 291–308.

Anderson, D.C. (2007) *Assessing the Human–Animal Bond*. Purdue University Press, West Lafayette, IN.

Anderson, E.C. (2004) Rinderpest. In *Bovine Medicine*, Andrews, A.H. (ed.), pp. 707–9. Blackwell Publishing, Oxford.

Andrews, A.H. (ed.) (2004) *Bovine Medicine*. Blackwell Publishing, Oxford.

Andrews, A.H. and Windsor, R.S. (2004) Respiratory conditions. In *Bovine Medicine*, Andrews, A.H. (ed.), pp. 860–74. Blackwell Publishing, Oxford.

Anonymous (1965) *Animal Health: a Centenary 1865–1965*. HMSO, London.

Anonymous (1999) *SAMM: Seasonal Approaches to Managing Mastitis*. Livestock Improvement Corporation, Hamilton.

Anonymous (2001a) *Basic Standards for Organic Production and Processing*. International Federation of Organic Agriculture Movements, Adelaide.

Anonymous (2001b) *Cost of Caring: Recognising Human Emotions in the Care of Laboratory Animals*. American Association for Laboratory Animal Science, Memphis, TN. www.aalas.org/pdf/06–00006.pdf.

Anonymous (2004) Welfare aspects of the castration of piglets. Scientific report of the panel for animal health and welfare on a request from the commission related to welfare aspects of the castration of piglets. *European Food Safety Authority Journal* **91**, 1–18.

Appleby, M.C., Mench, J.A. and Hughes, B.O. (2004) *Poultry Behaviour and Welfare.* CABI Publishing, Wallingford.

Archer, J. (1973) Tests for emotionality in rats and mice: a review. *Animal Behaviour* **21**, 205–35.

Arlinghaus, R., Cooke, S.J., Scwab A. and Cowx, I.G. (2007) Fish welfare: a challenge to the feelings-based approach, with implications for recreational fishing. *Fish and Fisheries* **8**, 57–71.

Arluke, A. (1992) Trapped in a guilt cage. *New Scientist* **134**, 33–5.

Baars, B.J. (2001) There are no known differences in brain mechanisms of consciousness between humans and other mammals. *Animal Welfare* **10**, S31–40.

Banner, M., Bulfield, G., Clark, S., Gormally, L., Hignett, P., Kimbell, H., Milburn, C. and Moffitt, J. (1995) *Report of the Committee to Consider the Ethical Implications of Emerging Technologies in the Breeding of Farm Animals.* HMSO, London.

Bantin, G.C. and Sanders, P.D. (1989) Animal caging: is bigger necessarily better? *Animal Technology* **40**, 45–54.

Barnard, C.J. and Hurst, J.L. (1996) Welfare by design: the natural selection of welfare criteria. *Animal Welfare* **5**, 405–33.

Barnett, J.L. and Hemsworth, P.H. (2003) Science and its application in assessing the welfare of laying hens. *Australian Veterinary Journal* **81**, 615–24.

Barnett, J.L., Hemsworth, P.H.J., Hennessy, D.P., McCallum, T.M. and Newman, E.A. (1994) The effects of modifying the amount of human contact on the behavioural, physiological and production responses of laying hens. *Applied Animal Behaviour Science* **41**, 87–100.

Bayvel, A.C.D. (2006) The international animal welfare role of the office international des epizooties: the world organisation for animal health. In *Animals, Ethics and Trade: The Challenge of Animal Sentience*, Turner, J. and D'Silva, J. (eds), pp. 248–60. Earthscan, London.

Beall, C.J., Phipps, A.J., Mathes, L.E., Stromberg, P. and Johnson, P.R. (2000) Transfer of the feline erythropoietin gene to cats using a recombinant adeno-associated virus vector. *Gene Therapy* **7**, 534–9.

Beausoleil, N.J., Blache, D., Stafford, K.J., Mellor, D.J. and Noble, A.D.L. (2008) Exploring the basis of divergent selection for 'temperament' in domestic sheep. *Applied Animal Behaviour Science* **109**, 261–74.

Benefiel, A.C. and Greenough, W.T. (1998) Effects of experience and environment on the developing and mature brain: implications for laboratory animal housing. *ILAR Journal* **39**, 5–11.

Benington, J.H. and Heller, H.C. (1995) Restoration of brain energy-metabolism as the function of sleep. *Progress in Neurobiology* **45**, 347–60.

Bennet, L., Rossenrode, S., Gunning, M.I., Gluckman, P.D. and Gunn, A.J. (1999) The cardiovascular and cerebrovascular responses of the immature fetal sheep to acute umbilical cord occlusion. *Journal of Physiology, London* **517**, 247–57.

Bennet, L., Westgate, J.A., Gluckman, P.D. and Gunn, A.J. (2003) Fetal responses to asphyxia. In *Neonatal Brain Injury: Mechanisms, Management, and the Risks of Practice*, Stevenson, D.K. and Sunshine, P. (eds), pp. 83–114. Cambridge University Press, Cambridge.

Berger, P.J., Walker, A.M., Horne, R., Brodecky, V., Wilkinson, M.H., Wilson, F. and Maloney, J.E. (1986) Phasic respiratory activity in the fetal lamb during late gestation and labour. *Respiratory Physiology* 65, 55–68.

Bingham, W.E. and. Griffiths, W.J., Jr. (1952) The effect of different environments during infancy on adult behavior in the rat. *Journal of Comparative and Physiological Psychology* 45, 307–12.

Blood, D.C. and Radostits, O.M. (1989) *Veterinary Medicine*. Bailliere Tindall, London.

Bonnet, M. (2005) Acute sleep deprivation. In *Principles and Practice of Sleep Medicine*, Kryger, M.H., Roth, T. and Dement, W.C. (eds), pp. 51–66. Elsevier Saunders, Philadelphia, PA.

Bradley, R.M. and Mistretta, C.M. (1975) Fetal sensory receptors. *Physiological Reviews* 55, 352–82.

Brambell, F.W.R. (1965) *Report of the Technical Committee to Enquire into the Welfare of Animals Kept Under Intensive Livestock Husbandry Systems*. HMSO, London.

Breuer, K., Hemsworth, P.H., Barnett, J.L., Matthews, L.R. and Coleman, G.J. (2000) Behavioural response to humans and the productivity of commercial dairy cows. *Applied Animal Behaviour Science* 66, 273–88.

Brightling, P., Mein, G.A., Malmo, J. and Ryan, D.P. (1998) *Countdown Downunder. Farm Guidelines for Mastitis Control*, pp. 1–122. Dairy Research and Development Corporation, Melbourne.

Broom, D.M. (1996) Animal welfare defined in terms of attempts of cope with the environment. *Acta agriculturae Scandinavica, Section A, Animal Science: Supplement* 27, 22–8.

Brown, J.P. and Silverman, J.P. (1999) The current and future market for veterinarians and veterinary medical services in the United States. *Journal of the American Veterinary Medical Association* 215, 161–83.

Brown, J.P., Cooper-Kuhn, C.M., Kempermann, G., van Praag, H., Winkler, J., Gage, F.H. and Kuhn, H.G. (2003) Enriched environment and physical activity stimulate hippocampal but not olfactory bulb neurogenesis. *European Journal of Neuroscience* 17, 2042–6.

Brown, R.T. (1968) Early experience and problem-solving ability. *Journal of Comparative and Physiological Psychology* 65, 433–40.

Calatayud, F., Belzung, C. and Aubert, A. (2004) Ethological validation and the assessment of anxiety-like behaviours: methodological comparison of classical analyses and structural approaches. *Behavioural Processes* 67, 195–206.

Carter, R. (1996) Holistic hazards. *New Scientist* 13 July, pp. 12–13. www.newscientist.com/article.ns?id=mg15120382.300.

Chamove, A.S. (1989) Cage design reduces emotionality in mice. *Laboratory Animals* 23, 215–19.

Chamove, A.S. (1994) Enrichment–past and future. *ANZCCART News* 7, 4–5.

Chamove, A.S., Anderson, J.R. and Nash, V.J. (1984) Social and environmental influences on self aggression in monkeys. *Primates* 25, 319–25.

Chapman, K., Abraham, C., Jenkins, V. and Fallowfield, L. (2003) Lay understanding of terms used in cancer consultations. *Psycho-Oncology* 12, 557–66.

Chesterton, R.N., Pfeiffer, D.U., Morris, R.S. and Tanner, C.M. (1989) Environmental and behavioural factors affecting the prevalence of foot lameness in New Zealand dairy herds – a case-control study. *New Zealand Veterinary Journal* 37, 135–52.

Clarkson, D.A. and Ward, W.R. (1991) Farm tracks, stockman's herding and lameness in dairy cattle. *Veterinary Record* 129, 511–12.

Conklin, A.R., Jr. and Stilwell, T.C. (2007) *World Food.* John Wiley and Sons, Hoboken, NJ.

Convery, I., Bailey, C., Mort, M. and Baxter, J. (2005) Death in the wrong place? Emotional geographies of the UK 2001 foot and mouth disease epidemic. *Journal of Rural Studies* 21, 99–109.

Crabbe, J.C., Wahlsten, D. and Dudek, B.C. (1999) Genetics of mouse behavior: interactions with laboratory environment. *Science* 284, 1670–72.

Curtis, J.W. and Nelson, C.A. (2003) Toward building a better brain: neurobehavioral outcomes, mechanisms, and processes of environmental enrichment. In *Resilence and Vulnerability: Adaptation in the Context of Childhood Adversities*, Luthar, S. (ed.), pp. 463–88. Cambridge University Press, London.

Davenport, J. (1976) Environmental therapy in hypothyroid and other disadvantaged animal populations. In *Environments as Therapy for Brain Dysfunction*, Walsh, R.N. and Greenough, W.T. (eds), pp. 71–114. Plenum Publishing Corporation, New York.

Davenport, J.W., Gonzalez, L.M., Carey, J.C., Bishop, S.B. and Hagquist, W.W. (1976) Environmental stimulation reduces learning deficits in experimental cretinism. *Science* 191, 578–9.

Davidson, R.M. (2002) Control and eradication of animal diseases in New Zealand. *New Zealand Veterinary Journal* 50, 6–12.

Davie, P.S. and Kopf, R.K. (2006) Physiology, behaviour and welfare of fish during recreational fishing and after release. *New Zealand Veterinary Journal* 54, 161–72.

Davis, J.H. (1987) Preadolescent self-concept development and pet ownership. *Anthrozoos*, 1, 90–4.

Dawkins, M.S. (1983) Battery hens name their price; consumer demand theory and the measurement of ethological needs. *Animal Behaviour* 31, 1195–1205.

Dawkins, M.S. (1998) Considering animal welfare from the animal's point of view. In *Responsible Conduct with Animals in Research*, Hart, L.A. (ed.), pp. 132–41. Oxford University Press, New York.

Deacon, R.M.J. (2006) Assessing nest building in mice. *Nature Protocols* 1, 1117–19.

de Bairacli Levy, J. (1953) *Herbal Handbook for Farm and Stable.* Faber and Faber, London.

Deboer, T. (1998) Brain temperature dependent changes in the electroencephalogram power spectrum of humans and animals. *Journal of Sleep Research* 7, 254–62.

Deboer, T. and Tobler, I. (1994) Sleep EEG after daily torpor in the Djungarian hamster: similarity to the effects of sleep deprivation. *Neuroscience Letters* 166, 35–8.

Dekkers, M. (2000) *Dearest Pet*. Verso, London.

DeLisi, L.E. (2001) Speech disorder in schizophrenia: review of the literature and exploration of its relation to the uniquely human capacity for language. *Schizophrenia Bulletin* 27, 481–96.

Denenberg, V.H. (1964) Critical periods, stimulus input, and emotional activity: a theory of infantile stimulation. *Psychological Review* 71, 335–51.

Denenberg, V.H. (1969) Open field behavior in the rat; what does it mean? *Annals of the New York Academy of Science* 159, 852–9.

Denenberg, V.H. and Morton, J.R.C. (1962) Effects of environmental complexity and social groupings upon modification of emotional behaviour. *Journal of Comparative and Physiological Psychology* 55, 242–6.

De Vries, A.C., Glasper, E.R. and Detillion, C.E. (2003) Social modulation of stress responses. *Physiology and Behavior* 79, 399–407.

Diamond, J. (2002) Evolution, consequences and future plant and animal domestication. *Nature* 418, 700–707.

Diesch, T.J., Mellor, D.J., Johnson, C.B. and Lentle, R.G. (2008) Responsiveness to painful stimuli in anaesthetised newborn and young animals of varying neurological maturity (wallaby joeys, rat pups and lambs). *AATEX Journal (Special Issue)* 14, 549–52.

Diesch, T.J., Mellor, D.J., Johnson, C.B. and Lentle, R.G. (2009) Electroencephalographic responses to tail clamping in anaesthetised rat pups aged 5 to 22 days. *Laboratory Animals* doi 10.1258/la.2008.0080083.

Doran, T. and Lambeth, L. (2007) Transforming livestock with transgenics: is designed resistance to viral diseases the way forward. In *Redesigning Animal Agriculture*, Swain, D.L., Charmley, E., Steel, J.W. and Coffey, S.G. (eds), pp. 121–43. CABI Publishing, Wallingford.

Duncan, I.J.H. (1981) Animal rights – animal welfare: a scientist's assessment. *Poultry Science* 60, 489–99.

Duncan, I.J.H. (1996) Animal welfare defined in terms of feelings. *Acta agriculturae Scandinavica, Section A, Animal Science: Supplement* 27, 29–35.

Duncan, I.J.H. (2005) Science-based assessment of animal welfare: farm animals. *Revue scientifique et technique, Office international des Epizooties* 24, 483–92.

Duncan, I.J.H. and Petherick, J.C. (1991) The implications of cognitive processes for animal welfare. *Journal of Animal Science* 69, 5017–22.

Duncan, I.J.H. and Olsson, I.A.S. (2001) Environmental enrichment: from flawed concept to pseudo-science. *Proceedings of the 35th International Congress of the International Society for Applied Ethology*, Davis, CA, p. 73 (abstract).

Dunlop, R.H. and Williams, D.J. (1996) Logic in the control of plagues and the understanding of diseases. In *History of Veterinary Medicine. Veterinary Medicine: an Illustrated History. Mosby Year Book, January*, pp. 277–90. Mosby-Year Book, St. Louis, MO.

Edney, A.T.B. (1998) Reasons for the euthanasia of dogs and cats. *Veterinary Record* 143, 114.

Einon, D. and Morgan, M. (1976) Habituation of object contact in socially reared and isolated rats (*Rattus norvergicus*). *Animal Behaviour* 24, 415–20.

Ellingson, R.J. and Rose, G.H. (1970) Ontogenesis of the electroencephalogram. In *Developmental Neurobiology*, Himwich, W.A. (ed), pp. 441–74. Charles C. Thomas Publisher, Springfield, IL.

Ellison, R.S. (2002) Major trace elements limiting livestock production in New Zealand. *New Zealand Veterinary Journal* 50, 35–40.

Evans, D.L. (2002) Welfare of the racehorse during exercise, training and racing. In *The Welfare of the Horse*, Waran, N. (ed.), pp. 180–201. Kluwer Academic Publishing, Dordrecht.

Ferguson, S.A., Racey, F.D., Paule, M.G. and Holson, R.R. (1993) Behavioral effects of methylazoxymethanol-induced microencephaly. *Behavioral Neuroscience* 107, 1067–76.

Fisher, M.W. and Mellor, D.J. (2002) The welfare implications of shepherding during lambing in extensive New Zealand farming systems. *Animal Welfare* 11, 157–70.

Fisher, M.W. and Mellor, D.J. (2008) Developing a systematic strategy incorporating ethical, animal welfare and practical principles to guide the genetic improvement of dairy cattle. *New Zealand Veterinary Journal* 65, 100–106.

Flannigan, G. and Dodman, N.H. (2001) Risk factors and behaviours associated with separation anxiety in dogs. *Journal of the American Veterinary Medical Association* 219, 460–66.

Flecknell, P.A. and Waterman-Pearson, A.E. (eds) (2000) *Pain Management in Animals.* WB Saunders, London.

Fowler, K.J., Sahhar, M.A. and Tassicker, R.J. (2000) Genetic counselling for cat and dog owners and breeders – managing the emotional impact. *Journal of the Veterinary Medical Association* 216, 498–501.

Fox, J. (1994) *Dairy Farmers 111 Ways to Improve Milking.* Fox Publications, Hamilton.

Fraser, A.F. and Broom, D.M. (1990) *Farm Animal Behaviour and Welfare*, pp. 198–207, 227–38. Beilliere Tindall, London.

Fraser, C. (2008) Disease risk to mozzarella output. *BBC News* 17 January. http://news.bbc.co.uk/2/hi/europe/7194281.stm.

Fraser, D. (2003) Assessing animal welfare at the farm and group level: the interplay of science and values. *Animal Welfare* 12, 433–43.

Fraser, D. (2008) Towards a global perspective on farm animal welfare. *Applied Animal Behaviour Science* 113, 330–39.

Fraser, D. and Duncan, I.J.H. (1998) "Pleasures", "pains" and animal welfare; towards a natural history of affect. *Animal Welfare* 7, 383–96.

Gallard, B.C., Peebles, C.M., Bolton, D.P.G. and Taylor, B.J. (1993) Sleep state organization in the developing piglet during exposure to different thermal stimuli. *Sleep* 16, 610–19.

Gentner, T.Q., Fenn, K.M., Margoliash, D. and Nusbaum, H.C. (2006) Recursive syntactic pattern learning by songbirds. *Nature* 440, 1204–7.

Giger, U., Sargan, D.R. and McNiel, E.A. (2006) Breed-specific hereditary diseases and genetic screening. In *The Dog and its Genome*, Cold Spring Harbor Monograph Series 44, Ostrander, E.A., Giger, U. and Lindblad-Toh, K. (eds), pp. 249–90. CSHL Press, Woodbury, NY.

Gill, J.H., Reid, L.D. and Porter, P.B. (1966) Effects of restricted rearing on Lashley stand performance. *Psychological Reports* 19, 239–42.

Gladwell, M. (2007) None of the above: what I.Q. doesn't tell you about race. *The New Yorker*, December 17.

Goddard, M.E. and Wiggans, G.R. (1999) Genetic improvement of dairy cattle. In *The Genetics of Cattle*, Fries, R. and Ruvinsky, A. (eds), pp. 511–38. CABI Publishing, Wallingford.

Gonyou, W.H. (1994) Why the study of animal behavior is associated with the animal welfare issue. *Journal of Animal Science* 72, 2171–7.

Gopal, R.M., West, D.M. and Pomroy, W.E. (2001) The difference in efficacy of ivermectin oral, moxidectin oral and moxidectin injectable formulations against an invermectin-resistant strain of *Trochostrongylus colubriformis*. *New Zealand Veterinary Journal* 49, 133–7.

Gosling, S.D. and John, O.P. (1999) Personality dimensions in nonhuman animals: a cross-species review. *Current Directions in Psychological Science* 8, 69–75.

Grandin, T. (1993) *Livestock Handling and Transport*. CABI Publishing, Wallingford.

Grandin, T. (1998) The feasibility of using vocalization scoring as an indicator of poor welfare during cattle slaughter. *Applied Animal Behaviour Science* 56, 121–8.

Grandin, T. and Deesing, M.J. (1998a) Genetics and behaviour during handling, restraint and herding. In *Genetics and the Behaviour of Domestic Animals*, Grandin, T. (ed.), pp. 113–44. Academic Press, San Diego, CA.

Grandin, T. and Deesing, M.J. (1998b) Genetics and animal welfare. In *Genetics and the Behaviour of Domestic Animals*, Grandin, T. (ed.), pp. 319–46. Academic Press, San Diego, CA.

Green, R.E., Corness, S.J., Scharlemann, J.P.W. and Balmford, A. (2005) Farming and the fate of nature. *Science* 307, 550–55.

Gregory, N.G. (1998) Physiological mechanisms causing sickness behaviour and suffering in diseased animals. *Animal Welfare* 7, 293–305.

Gregory, N.G. (2004) *Physiology and Behaviour of Animal Suffering*. UFAW Animal Welfare Series, pp. 1–11. Blackwell Publishing, Oxford.

Guthrie, R.V. (1998) *Even the Rat was White*. Allyn and Bacon, Needham Heights, MA.

Gvaryahu, G. and Snapir, N. (1997) Contact lenses for laying hens. *Journal of Applied Poultry Research* 6, 449–52.

Hall, C.S. (1934) Emotional behavior in the rat. I Defaecation and urination as measures of individual differences in emotionality. *Journal of Comparative and Physiological Psychology* 18, 385–403.

Hamilton, C., Hansson, I., Ekman, T., Emanuelson, U. and Forslund, K. (2002) Health of cows, calves and young stock on 26 organic herds in Sweden. *Veterinary Record* 150, 503–8.

Hand, M.S., Thatcher, C.D., Remillard, R.L. and Roudebush, P. (2000) *Small Animal Clinical Nutrition*. Mark Morris Institute, Topeka, KA.

Hanninen, L. (2007) *Sleep and Rest in Calves: Relationship to Welfare, Housing and Hormonal Activity*. Academic dissertation, Department of Production Animal Medicine, Faculty of Veterinary Medicine, University of Helsinki, Helsinki.

Harlow, H.F. (1959) Love in infant monkeys. *Scientific American* 200, 68–74.

Hasan, S.U. and Rigaux, A. (1991) The effects of lung distension, oxygenation, and gestational age on fetal behavior and breathing movements in sheep. *Pediatric Research* 30, 193–201.

Haslam, N. (2006) Dehumanisation: an integrative review. *Personality and Social Psychology* 10, 252–64.

Hebb, D. (1949) *The Organization of Behavior*. Wiley, New York.

Heller, H.C. and Ruby, N.F. (2004) Sleep and circadian rhythms in mammalian torpor. *Annual Review of Physiology* 66, 275–89.

Hemsworth, P.H. and Barnett, J.L. (1987) Human–animal interactions. *Veterinary Clinics of North America: Food Animal Practice* 3, 339–56.

Hemsworth, P.H.J. and Coleman, G.J. (1998) *Human–Livestock Interactions*. CABI Publishing, Wallingford.

Hennessy, M.B., David, H.N., Williams, M.T., Mellott, C. and Douglas, C.W. (1997) Plasma cortisol levels of dogs at a county animal shelter. *Physiology and Behaviour* 62, 485–90.

Herzog, H. (2002) Ethical aspects of relationships between humans and research animals. *ILAR Journal* 43, 27–32.

Hickey, M.C., French, P. and Grant, J. (2002) Out-wintering pads for finishing beef cattle: animal production and welfare. *Animal Science* 75, 447–58.

Holloway, R.L., Jr. (1966) Dendritic branching: some preliminary results of training and complexity in rat visual cortex. *Brain Research* 2, 393–6.

Holmes, C.W., Brookes, I.M., Garick, D.J., Mackenzie, D.D.S., Parkinson, T.J. and Wilson, G.F. (2002) *Milk Production from Pasture*. Massey University, Palmerston North.

Holson, R.R. (1986) Feeding neophobia: a possible explanation for the differential maze performance for the rats reared in enriched or isolated environments. *Physiology and Behaviour* 38, 191–201.

Hsu, Y., Severinghaus, L.L. and Serpell, J.A. (2003) Dog keeping in Taiwan: its contribution to the problem of free-roaming dogs. *Journal of Applied Animal Welfare Science* 6, 1–23.

Hunter, C.J., Bennet, L., Power, G.G., Roelfsema, V., Blood, A.B., Quaedackers, J.S., George, S., Guan, J. and Gunn, A.J. (2003) Key neuroprotective role for endogenous adenosine A_1 receptor activation during asphyxia in the fetal sheep. *Stroke* 34, 2240–45.

Hymovitch, B. (1952) The effects of experimental variations on problem solving in the rat. *Journal of Comparative and Physiological Psychology* 45, 313–21.

Iliff, S.A. (2002) An additional "R": remembering the animals. *ILAR Journal* 43, 38–47.

Irvin, D. (2007) Control debate, growers advised. *Arkansas Democrat Gazette*, 2 December. www.nwanews.com/adg/Business/202171/.

Johnson, C.B., Sylvester, S.P., Stafford, K.J., Mitchinson, S.L., Ward, R.N. and Mellor, D.J. (2009) Effects of age on the electroencephalographic response to castration in lambs anaesthetised using halothane in oxygen from birth to six weeks old. *Veterinary Anaesthesia and Analgesia* 36, 273–9.

Jolly, R.D. (2002) Mannosidosis in cattle and its control. *New Zealand Veterinary Journal* 50, 90.

Jones, A.C. and Gosling, S.D. (2005) Temperament and personality in dogs (Canis familiaris): a review and evaluation of past research. *Applied Animal Behaviour Research* **95**, 1–53.

Jule, K.R., Leaver, L.A. and Lea, E.G. (2008) The effects of captive experience on reintroduction survival in carnivores: a review and analysis. *Biological Conservation* **141**, 355–63.

Kaminski, J., Riedel, J., Call, J. and Tomasello, M. (2005) Domestic goats, *Capra hircus*, follow gaze direction and use social cues in a object choice task. *Animal Behaviour* **69**, 11–18.

Karmanova, I.G. (1982) *Evolution of Sleep: Stages of the Formation of the 'Wakefulness-Sleep' Cycle in Vertebrates*, pp. 1–164. S. Karger AG, Basel.

Kellert, S.R. (1988) Human animal interactions: a review of American attitudes to wild and domestic animals in the twentieth century. In *Animals and People Sharing the World*, Rowan, A.N. (ed.), pp. 137–75. University Press of New England, NH.

Kempermann, G., Kuhn, H.G. and Gage, F.H. (1997) More hippocampal neurons in adult mice living in an enriched environment. *Nature*, **386**, 493–5.

Kendrick, K.M. (2007) Quality of life and the evolution of the brain. *Animal Welfare* **16(S)**, 9–15.

Kidd, A.H., Kidd, R.M. and George, C.G. (1992) Successful and unsuccessful pet adoptions. *Psychological Reports* **70**, 547–61.

Kilgour, R. (1971) Animal handling in works: pertinent behaviour studies. In *Proceedings of the 13th Meat Industry Research Conference*, Hamilton, New Zealand, pp. 9–12.

Kilgour, R. and Dalton, C. (1984) *Livestock Behaviour: a Practical Guide*. Methuen, Auckland.

Kirkwood, J.K. (2006) The distribution of the capacity for sentience in the animal kingdom. In *Animals, Ethics and Trade: the Challenge of Animal Sentience*, Turner, J. and D'Silva, J. (eds), pp. 12–26. Earthscan, London.

Kirkwood, J.K., Hubrecht, R.C., Wickens, S., O'Leary, H. and Oakeley, S. (eds) (2001) Consciousness, cognition and animal welfare. *Animal Welfare* **10** (suppl.), S1–251.

Kirkwood, J.K., Roberts, E.A. and Vickery, S. (eds) (2004) Science in the service of animal welfare. *Animal Welfare* **13** (suppl.), S1–259.

Kitching, R.P. (2004) Foot-and-mouth disease. In *Bovine Medicine*, Andrews, A.H. (ed.), pp. 700–706. Blackwell Publishing, Oxford.

Kobelt, A.J. (2004) *The behaviour and Welfare of Pet Dogs in Suburban Backyards*. PhD thesis, University of Melbourne, Victoria.

Koene, P. and Duncan, I.J.H. (2001) From environmental requirement to environmental enrichment: from animal suffering to animal pleasure. *Proceedings of the Fifth International Conference on Environmental Enrichment*, 4–9 November 2001, Sydney, Australia, p. 205.

Kolb, B. and Elliott, W. (1987) Recovery from early cortical damage in rats. II. Effects of experience on anatomy and behavior following frontal lesions at 1 or 5 days of age. *Behavioural Brain Research* **26**, 47–56.

Kortner, G. and Geiser, F. (2000) The temporal organization of daily torpor and hibernation: circadian and circannual rhythms. *Chronobiology International* **17**, 103–28.

Kulpa-Eddy, J.A., Taylor, S. and Adams, K.M. (2005) USDA perspective on environmental enrichment for animals. *ILAR Journal* 46, 83–94.

Kyriazakis, I. and Whittemore, C.T. (2006) *Whittemore's Science and Practice of Pig Production*. Blackwell Publishing, Oxford.

Lacheretz, A., Moreau, D. and Cathelain, H. (2002) Causes of death and life expectancy in carnivorous pets (I). *Revue de Medecine Veterinaire* 153, 819–22.

Lautenbacher, S., Kundermann, B. and Krieg, J.-C. (2006) Sleep deprivation and pain perception. *Sleep Medicine Reviews* 10, 357–69.

Lee, S.J., Peter Ralston, H.J., Drey, E.A., Partridge, J.C. and Rosen, M.A. (2005) Fetal pain: a systematic multidisciplinary review of the evidence. *Journal of the American Medical Association* 294, 947–54.

Leslie, B.E., Meek, A.H., Kawash, G.F. and McKeown, D.B. (1994) An epidemiological survey of pet ownership in Ontario. *Canadian Veterinary Journal* 35, 218–22.

Levine, S. (1960) Anoxic-ischemic encephalopathy in rats. *American Journal of Pathology* 36, 1–17.

Lima, S.L., Rattenborg, N.C., Lesku, J.A. and Amlaner, C.J. (2005) Sleeping under the risk of predation. *Animal Behaviour* 70, 723–6.

Linde-Forsberg, C. (2001) Reproduction and modern reproductive technology. In *The Genetics of the Dog*, Ruvinsky, A. and Sampson. J. (eds), pp. 461–85. CABI Publishing, Wallingford.

Lloyd, J.K.F. (2004) *Exploring the Match Between People and their Guide Dogs*. PhD thesis, Massey University, Palmerston North.

Lund, V. and Olsson, I.A.S. (2005) Animal agriculture: symbiosis, culture, or ethical conflict? *Journal of Agricultural and Environmental Ethics* 19, 47–56.

Lynch, J.J. and Gantt, W. (1968) The heart rate component of the social reflex in dogs: the conditional effect of petting and person. *Conditioned Reflex* 3, 69–80.

Mackay, A.D. (2001) Non-chemical farming: overview and practicalities. *Proceedings of the 31st Seminar of the Society of Sheep and Beef Cattle Veterinarians of the New Zealand Veterinary Association*, pp. 51–60. Foundation for Continuing Veterinary Education of the New Zealand Veterinary Association, Massey University, Palmerston North.

MacLeod, G. (1964) *The Treatment of Cattle by Homeopathy*. Health Science Press, Essex.

Mallard, E.C., Gunn, A.J., Williams, C.E., Johnston, B.M. and Gluckman, P.D. (1992) Transient umbilical cord occlusion causes hippocampal damage in the fetal sheep. *American Journal Obstetrics Gynecology* 167, 1423–30.

Markel, A.L., Galaktionov, Yu.K. and Efimov, V.M. (1999) Factor analysis of rat behavior in an open field test. *Neuroscience and Behavioral Physiology* 19, 279–86.

Markowitz, H. (1982) *Behavioral Enrichment in the Zoo*. Van Nostrand Reinhold, New York.

Markowitz, H. and Line, S. (1990) The need for responsive environments. In *The Experimental Animal in Biomedical Research*, Rollin, B.E. (ed.), vol. I, pp. 152–70. CRC Press, Boca Raton, FL.

Markowitz, H. and Aday, C. (1998) Power for captive animals: contingencies and nature. In *Second Nature: Environmental Enrichment for Captive Animals*,

Shepherdson, D.J., Mellen, J.D. and Hutchins, M. (eds), Smithsonian Institution Press, Washington DC.

Martin, J. (2000) *The Development of Modern Agriculture*. Macmillan Press, Basingstoke.

Marx, G., Horn, T., Thielebein, J., Knubel, B. and von Borell, E. (2003) Analysis of pain-related vocalization in young pigs. *Journal of Sound and Vibration* 266, 687–98.

Mason, T.A. and Bourke, J.M. (1973) Closure of the distal radial epiphysis and its relationship to unsoundness in two year old thoroughbreds. *Australian Veterinary Journal* 49, 221–8.

McDonald, P., Small, A. and Wales, W.J. (1994) Animal production, nutrition and health of biodynamic compared to conventional dairy cattle. *Proceedings of International Federation of Organic Agriculture Movements*, Lincoln University, Canterbury, p. 105.

McGlone, J. and Pond, W. (2003) *Pig Production: Biological Principles and Applications*. Thomson/Delmar Learning, New York.

McGreevy, P.D. and Nicholas, F.W. (1999) Some practical solutions to welfare problems in dog breeding. *Animal Welfare* 8, 329–41.

McInerney, J.P. (1998) The economics of welfare. In *Ethics, Welfare, Law and Market Forces: the Veterinary Interface*, Michell, A.R. and Edwards, R. (eds), Proceedings of a Royal College of Veterinary Surgeons (RCVS) and Universities Federation of Animal Welfare (UFAW) Symposium, November 1996, pp. 115–34. UFAW, London.

Meddis, R. (1975) On the function of sleep. *Animal Behaviour* 23, 676–91.

Mehlman, B. (1967) Animal research and human psychology. *Journal of Humanistic Psychology* 7, 66–79.

Mellen, J. and MacPhee, M.S. (2001) Philosophy of environmental enrichment: past, present, and future. *Zoo Biology* 20, 211–26.

Mellor, D.J. (1998) How can animal-based scientists demonstrate ethical integrity? In *Ethical Approaches to Animal-Based Science*, Mellor, D.J., Fisher, M. and Sutherland, G. (eds), pp. 19–31. Australian and New Zealand Council for the Care of Animals in Research and Teaching, Royal Society of New Zealand, Wellington.

Mellor, D.J. (2003) Guidelines for the humane slaughter of the fetuses of pregnant ruminants. *Surveillance* 30, 26–8.

Mellor, D.J. (2004a) Comprehensive assessment of harms caused by experimental, teaching and testing procedures on live animals. *Alternatives of Laboratory Animals* 32 (suppl. 1), 453–7.

Mellor, D.J. (2004b) Chairman's comment: "Good practice" and "scientific knowledge" and their application to setting minimum standards. *National Animal Welfare Advisory Committee 2003 Annual Report*, pp. 4–8. Ministry of Agriculture and Forestry, Wellington.

Mellor, D.J. and Reid, C.S.W. (1994) Concepts of animal well-being and predicting the impact of procedures on experimental animals. In *Improving the Well-Being of Animals in the Research Environment*, Baker, R.M., Jenkin, G., and Mellor, D.J. (eds), pp. 3–18. Australian and New Zealand Council for the Care of Animals in Research and Teaching, Glen Osmond, South Australia.

Mellor, D.J. and Battye, J. (2000) Making a profession of science; the two-way street of public trust and concern for public good. In *Ethical Approaches to Animal-Based Science*,

Mellor, D.J., Fisher, M. and Sutherland, G. (eds), pp. 125–33. Australian and New Zealand Council for the Care of Animals in Research and Teaching, Royal Society of New Zealand, Wellington.

Mellor, D.J. and Stafford, K.J. (2000) Acute castration and tailing distress and its alleviation in lambs. *New Zealand Veterinary Journal* 48, 33–43.

Mellor, D.J. and Stafford, K.J. (2001) Integrating practical, regulatory and ethical strategies for enhancing farm animal welfare. *Australian Veterinary Journal* 79, 762–8.

Mellor, D.J. and Gregory, N.G. (2003) Responsiveness, behavioural arousal and awareness in fetal and newborn lambs: experimental, practical and therapeutic implications. *New Zealand Veterinary Journal* 51, 2–13.

Mellor, D.J and Battye, J. (2004) Mutual respect overcomes mutual disregard: working to resolve the GE impasse. In *Reflections on the Use of Human Genes in Other Organisms: Ethical, Spiritual and Cultural Dimensions*, pp. 15–19. The Bioethics Council, Ministry for the Environment, Wellington.

Mellor, D.J. and Bayvel, A.C.D. (2004) Application of legislation, scientific guidelines and codified standards for advancing animal welfare. *Global Conference on Animal Welfare: an OIE Initiative*, Proceedings of an OIE Conference, Paris, France, 23–25 February, pp. 249–59.

Mellor, D.J. and Stafford, K.J. (2004) Animal welfare implications of neonatal mortality and morbidity in farm animals. *Veterinary Journal* 168, 118–33.

Mellor, D.J. and Diesch, T.J. (2006) Onset of sentience: the potential for suffering in fetal and newborn farm animals. *Applied Animal Behaviour Science* 100, 48–57.

Mellor, D.J. and Diesch, T.J. (2007) Birth and hatching: key events in the onset of 'awareness' in lambs and chicks. *New Zealand Veterinary Journal* 55, 51–60.

Mellor, D.J. and Bayvel, A.C.D. (2008) New Zealand's inclusive science-based system for setting animal welfare standards. *Applied Animal Behaviour Science* 113, 313–29.

Mellor, D.J., Cook, C.J. and Stafford, K.J. (2000) Chapter 9: Quantifying some responses to pain as a stressor. In *The Biology of Animal Stress: Basic Principles and Implications for Welfare*, Moberg, G.P. and Mench, J.A. (eds), pp. 171–98. CABI Publishing, Wallingford.

Mellor, D.J., Diesch, T.J., Gunn, A.J. and Bennet, L. (2005) The importance of 'awareness' for understanding fetal pain. *Brain Research Reviews* 49, 455–71.

Mellor, D.J., Diesch, T.J., Gunn, A.J. and Bennet, L. (2008a) Fetal 'awareness' and 'pain': what precautions should be taken to safeguard fetal welfare during experiments? *AATEX Journal (Special Issue)* 14, 79–83.

Mellor, D.J., Thornber, P.M., Bayvel, A.C.D. and Kahn, S. (eds) (2008b) Scientific assessment and management of animal pain. *OIE Technical Series* 10, 1–218.

Mendl, M. and Paul, E.S. (2004) Consciousness, emotion and animal welfare: insights from cognitive science. *Animal Welfare* 13, 17–25.

Mepham, B. (2000) A framework for the ethical analysis of novel foods: the ethical matrix. *Journal of Agricultural and Environmental Ethics* 12, 165–76.

Miglior, F., Muir, B.L. and Van Doormaal, B.J. (2005) Selection indices in Holstein cattle of various countries. *Journal of Dairy Science* 88, 1255–63.

Miklosi, A., Kubinti, E., Topal, J., Gacsi, M., Viranyi, Z. and Csanyi, V. (2003) A simple reason for a big difference: wolves do not look back at humans, but dogs do. *Current Biology* **13**, 763–6.

Morgan, M.J. (1973) Effects of postweaning environment of learning in the rat. *Animal Behaviour* **21**, 429–42.

Morton, D.B. and Griffiths, P.H. (1985) Guidelines on the recognition of pain, distress and discomfort in experimental animals and an hypothesis for assessment. *Veterinary Record* **116**, 431–6.

Morton, E.S. (1977) On the occurrence and significance of motivation structural rules in some bird and mammal sounds. *American Naturalist* **3**, 855–69.

Mullins, M.H. (1999) Mirrors and windows: sociocultural studies of human–animal relationships. *Annual Review of Anthropology* **28**, 201–24.

Munro, H.M.C. and Thrusfield, M.V. (2001a) 'Battered pets': features that raise suspicion of non-accidental injury. *Journal of Small Animal Practice* **42**, 218–26.

Munro, H.M.C. and Thrusfield, M.V. (2001b) 'Battered pets': injuries found in dogs and cats. *Journal of Small Animal Practice* **42**, 279–90.

Munro, H.M.C. and Thrusfield, M.V. (2001c) 'Battered pets': sexual abuse. *Journal of Small Animal Practice* **42**, 333–7.

Munro, H.M.C. and Thrusfield, M.V. (2001d) 'Battered pets': Munchausen syndrome by proxy (factitious illness by proxy). *Journal of Small Animal Practice* **42**, 385–9.

Newberry, R.C. (1995) Environmental enrichment: increasing the biological relevance of captive environments. *Applied Animal Behavioural Science* **44**, 229–43.

Newton, R. and Chanter, N. (2003) Strangles. In *Current Therapy in Equine Medicine*, Robinson, N.E. (ed.), pp. 64–68. Saunders, Philadelphia, PA.

Nicholas, F.W. (1996) *Introduction to Veterinary Genetics*. Oxford University Press, Oxford.

Nielsen, N. (1992) Ecosystem health and veterinary medicine. *Canadian Veterinary Journal* **33**, 23–6.

Nordenfelt, L. (2006) *Animal and Human Health and Welfare: a Comparative Philosophical Analysis*. CABI Publishing, Wallingford.

Oberbauer, A.M. and Sampson, J. (2001) Pedigree analysis and genetic counselling. In *The Genetics of the Dog*, Ruvinsky, A. and Sampson, J. (eds), pp. 461–85. CABI Publishing, Wallingford.

Odendaal, J.S.J. and Meintjes, R.A. (2003) Neurophysiological correlates of affiliative behaviour between humans and dogs. *Veterinary Journal* **165**, 296–301.

Overall, K.L. (1997) *Clinical Behavioral Medicine for Small Animals*. Mosby, St. Louis, MO.

Padgett, G.A. (1998) *Control of Canine Genetic Diseases*. Howell Book House, New York.

Parsons, P.J. and Spear, N.E. (1972) Long-term retention of avoidance learning by immature and adult rats as a function of environmental enrichment. *Journal of Comparative and Physiological Psychology* **80**, 297–303.

Patterson-Kane, E.G. (1999) *Assessing and Enriching the Cage Environment of Laboratory Rats*. PhD thesis, Victoria University of Wellington, Wellington.

Paulson, I. (1964) The animal guardian: a critical and synthetic review. *History of Religions* 3, 202–19.

Pepperberg, I.M. (1987) Evidence for conceptual quantitative abilities in the African grey parrot: labeling of cardinal sets. *Ethology* 75, 37–61.

Perkins, N.R., Reid, S.W.J. and Morris, R.S. (2005) Risk factors for musculoskeletal injuries of the lower limbs in thoroughbred racehorses in New Zealand. *New Zealand Veterinary Journal* 53, 171–83.

Phipps, N.M. (2003) *Rehoming Animals from Animal Rescue Shelters in New Zealand.* MSc thesis, Massey University.

Pond, W.G., Church, D.C., Pond, K.R. and Schoknecht, P.A. (2004) *Basic Animal Nutrition and Feeding.* Wiley, Hoboken, NJ.

Poole, T. (1997) Happy animals make good science. *Lab Animals* 31, 116–24.

Porter, V. (1991) *Cattle: a Handbook to the Breeds of the World.* The Crowood Press, Wiltshire.

Premack, D. (2004) Is language the key to human intelligence? *Science* 303, 318–20.

Price, E.O. (2002) *Animal Domestication and Behaviour.* CABI Publishing, Wallingford.

Prut, L. and Belzung, C. (2003) The open-field as a paradigm to measure effects of drugs on anxiety-like behaviours: a review. *European Journal of Pharmacology* 463, 3–33.

Purves, K.E. (1997) Rat and mice enrichment. In *Animal Alternatives, Welfare and Ethics,* Van Zutphen, L.F.M. and Balls, M. (eds), *Proceedings of the 2nd World Congress on Alternatives and Animal Use in the Life Sciences,* Utrecht, The Netherlands, pp. 199–207.

Rasmussen, J.L. and Rajecki, D.W. (1995) Differences and similarities in humans' perceptions of the thinking and feeling of a dog and a boy. *Society and Animals* 3, 117–37.

Rattenborg, N.C., Amlaner, C.J. and Lima, S.L. (2000) Behavioural, neurophysiological and evolutionary perspectives on unihemispheric sleep. *Neuroscience and Biobehavioral Reviews* 24, 817–42.

Rauscher, F.H. and Zupan, M. (2000) Classroom keyboard instruction improves kindergarten children's spatial-temporal performance: a field experiment. *Early Childhood Research Quarterly* 15, 215–28.

Rauscher, F.H., Shaw, G.L. and Ky, K.N. (1995) Listening to Mozart enhances spatialtemporal reasoning: towards a neurophysiological basis. *Neuroscience Letters* 185, 44–7.

Rauscher, F.H. , Robinson, K.D. and Jens, J. (1998) Improved maze learning through early music exposure in rats. *Neurological Research* 20, 427–32.

Renner, M. and Rosenzweig, M. (1987) *Enriched and Impoverished Environments.* Springer-Verlag, New York.

Robertson, A. (1976) *Handbook of Animal Diseases in the Tropics.* British Veterinary Association, London.

Robinson, I. (1995) *The Waltham Book of Human–Animal Interaction.* Pergamon, Elsevier Science, Oxford.

Robinson, N.E. (2003) *Current Therapy in Equine Medicine.* Saunders, Philadelphia, PA.

Roeder, J.J., Chetecuti, Y. and Will, B. (1980) Behavior and length of survival of populations of enriched and impoverished rats in the presence of a predator. *Biology of Behavior* 5, 361–9.

Rogers, L.J. (1995) Comparison with development in other species. In *The Development of Brain and Behaviour in the Chicken*, pp. 184–212. CABI Publishing, Wallingford.

Rogers, P. and Janssens, L. (1991) Acupuncture in animals. *Proceedings of the Post-Graduate Committee in Veterinary Science*, No. 167, University of Sydney, Sydney, pp. 1–548.

Rollin, B. (1992) *Animal Rights and Human Morality*. Prometheus Books, Buffalo, NY.

Rollin, B. (1995) *Farm Animal Welfare: Social, Bioethical and Research Issues*. Iowa State University Press, Ames, IO.

Rose, F.D. (1988) Environmental enrichment and recovery of function following brain damage in the rat. *Medical Science Research* **16**, 257–63.

Rose, F.D., Dell, P.A. and Love. S. (1987) An analysis of reinforcement in rats reared in enriched and impoverished environments. *Medical Science Research: Psychology and Psychiatry* **15**, 717–18.

Rosenzweig, M.R. and Bennett, E.L. (1972) Cerebral changes in rats exposed individually to an enriched environment. *Journal of Comparative Physiology and Psychology* **80**, 304–13.

Rosenzweig, M.R., Bennett, E.L. and Diamond, M.C. (1972) Brain changes in response to experience. *Scientific American* **226**, 22–9.

Ruckebusch, Y. (1974) Sleep deprivation in cattle. *Brain Research* **78**, 495–9.

Ruckebusch, Y. (1975) The hypnogram as an index of adaptation of farm animals to changes in their environment. *Applied Animal Ethology* **2**, 3–18.

Ruis, M.A.W., te Brake, J.H.A., van de Burgwal, J.A., de Jong, I.C., Blokhuis, H.J. and Koolhaas, J.M. (2000) Personalities in female domesticated pigs: behavioural and physiological indications. *Applied Animal Behaviour Science* **66**, 31–47.

Rushen, J. (2008) Farm animal welfare since the Brambell report. *Applied Animal Behaviour Science* **113**, 277–8.

Rushen, J., Taylor, A.A. and de Passille, A.M. (1999) Domestic animals' fear of humans and its effect on their welfare. *Applied Animal Behaviour Science* **65**, 285–303.

Russow, L.-M. (2002) Ethical implications of the human–animal bond in the laboratory. *ILAR Journal* **43**, 33–43.

Ryan, O. (2006) Animal welfare and economic development: a financial institution perspective. In *Animals, Ethics and Trade: The Challenge of Animal Sentience*, Turner, J. and D'Silva, J. (eds), pp. 238–47. Earthscan, London.

Ryder, R.D. (1998) Painism. *Encyclopedia of Applied Ethics*, vol. 3, pp. 415–18. Academic Press, New York.

Scanes, C.G., Brant, G. and Ensminger, M.E. (2004) *Poultry Science*. Pearson/Prentice Hall, Upper Saddle River, NJ.

Schroder, M.J.A. and McEachern, M.G. (2004) Consumer value conflicts surrounding ethical food purchase decisions: a focus on animal welfare. *International Journal of Consumer Studies* **28**, 168.

Scobie, D.R., Bray, A.R. and O'Connell, D. (1999) A breeding goal to improve the welfare of sheep. *Animal Welfare* **8**, 391–406.

Scott, E.M., Fitzpatrick, J.L., Nolan, A.M., Reid, J. and Wiseman, M.L. (2003) Evaluation of welfare state based on interpretation of multiple indices. *Animal Welfare* **12**, 457–68.

Seabrook, M.F. (1972) A study to determine the influence of the herdsman's personality on milk yield. *Journal of Agriculture Labour Science* 1, 45–59.

Serpell, J.A. (1999) Sheep in wolf's clothing? Attitudes to animals among farmers and scientists. In *Attitudes to Animals: Views in Animal Welfare*, Dolins, F.L. (ed.), pp. 26–33. Cambridge University Press, Cambridge.

Serpell, J.A. (2005) Factors influencing veterinary students' career choices and attitudes to animals. *Journal of Veterinary Medical Education* 32, 491–6.

Shapiro, C.M. and Flanigan, M.J. (1993) ABC of sleep disorders. Function of sleep. *British Medical Journal* 306, 383–5.

Shaw, J. (2007) *World Food Security*. Palgrave Macmillan, Basingstoke.

Siegel, J.M. (2005) Clues to the functions of mammalian sleep. *Nature* 437, 1264–71.

Simmonds, M.P. (2006) Into the brains of whales. *Applied Animal Behaviour Science* 100, 103–16.

Singer, P. (1990) *Animal Liberation*, 2nd edn. New York Review of Books, New York.

Smidt, D. and Niemann, H. (1999) Biotechnology in genetics and reproduction. *Livestock Production Science* 59, 207–21.

Smith, B.L. and Towers, N.R. (2002) Mycotoxicosis of grazing animals in New Zealand. *New Zealand Veterinary Journal* 50, 28–34.

Smith, C. (1985) Sleep states and learning: a review of the animal literature. *Neuroscience and Biobehavioral Reviews* 9, 157–68.

Smith, H.V. (1972) Effects of environmental enrichment on open-field activity and Hebb-Williams problem solving in rats. *Journal of Comparative and Physiological Psychology* 80, 163–168.

Snead, O.C. and Stephens, H.I. (1983) Ontogeny of cortical and subcortical electroencephalographic events in unrestrained neonatal and infant rats. *Experimental Neurology* 82, 249–69.

Soskin, R.A. (1963) The effect of early experience upon the formation of environmental preferences in rats. *Journal of Comparative and Physiological Psychology* 56, 303–6.

Spedding, C. (2000) *Animal Welfare*, pp. 31–44. Earthscan, London.

Spence, F.T. and Maher, B.A. (1962) Handling and noxious stimulation of the albino rat. II effects on subsequent performance in a learning situation. *Journal of Comparative and Physiological Psychology* 55, 252–5.

Spinka, M., Newberry, R.C. and Bekoff, M. (2001) Mammalian play: training for the unexpected. *Quarterly Review of Biology* 76, 141–68.

Spires, T.L., Grote, H.E., Varshney, N.K., Cordery, P.M., van Dellen, A., Blakemore, C. and Hannan, A. (2004) Environmental enrichment rescues protein deficits in a mouse model of Huntington's Disease, indicating a possible disease mechanism. *Journal of Neuroscience* 24, 2270–76.

Stafford, K.J. (1989) Animal health and production in the Tihama area of the Yemen Arab Republic. *Tropicultura* 7, 172–4.

Stafford, K. (2006) *The Welfare of Dogs*. Springer, Dordrecht.

Stafford, K.J. and Mellor, D.J. (2005a) The welfare significance of the castration of cattle: a review. *New Zealand Veterinary Journal* 53, 271–8.

Stafford, K.J. and Mellor, D.J. (2005b) Dehorning and disbudding distress and its alleviation in calves. *Veterinary Journal* 169, 337–49.

Stewart, M.F. (2001) *Companion Animal Death.* Butterworth Heinemann, Oxford.

Stickgold, R. (2005) Sleep-dependent memory consolidation. *Nature* 437, 1272–8.

Stricklin, W.R. (1995) Space as environmental enrichment. *Lab Animal* 24, 24.

Swaisgood, R.R. and Shepherdson, D.J. (2005) Scientific approaches to enrichment and stereotypies in zoo animals: what's been done and where should we go next? *Zoo Biology* 24, 499–518.

Taylor, A.A. and Weary, D.M. (2000) Vocal responses of piglets to castration: identifying procedural sources of pain. *Applied Animal Behaviour Science* 70, 17–26.

Tellam, R. (2007) The impact of genomics on livestock production. In *Redesigning Animal Agriculture*, Swain, D.L., Charmley, E., Steel, J.W. and Coffey, S.G. (eds), pp. 46–64. CABI Publishing, Wallingford.

Tilman, D., Cassman, K.G., Matson, P.A., Naylor, R. and Polasky, S. (2002) Agricultural sustainability and intensive production practices. *Nature* 418, 671–7.

Toth, L.A. (1995) Sleep, sleep deprivation and infectious diseases: studies in animals. *Advances in Neuroimmunology* 5, 79–92.

Trewavas, A. (2002) Malthus foiled again and again. *Nature* 418, 668–70.

Trut, L.N. (1999) Early canid domestication: the farm-fox experiment. *American Scientist* 87, 160–69.

Tung, A. and Mendelson, W.B. (2004) Anesthesia and sleep. *Sleep Medicine Reviews* 8, 213–25.

Turner, J. and D'Silva, J. (eds) (2006) *Animals, Ethics and Trade: The Challenge of Animal Sentience.* Earthscan, London.

Tyndale-Biscoe, C.H. and Janssens, P.A. (eds) (1988) *The Developing Marsupial: Models for Biomedical Research.* Springer-Verlag, Heidelberg.

van der Staay, F.J. and Steckler, T. (2002) The fallacy of behavioural phenotyping without standardization. *Genes, Brain and Behavior* 1, 9–13.

van der Valk, J., Mellor, D., Brands, R., Fischer, R., Gruber, F., Gstraunthaler, G., Hellebrekers, L., Hyllner, J., Jonker, H., Prieto, P. *et al.* (2004) The humane collection of fetal bovine serum and possibilities for serum-free cell and tissue culture. *Toxicology In Vitro* 18, 1–12.

Van Loo, P.L.P. and Baumans, V. (2004) The importance of learning young: the use of nesting material in laboratory rats. *Laboratory Animals* 38, 17–24.

van Praag, H., Kempermann, G. and Gage, F.H. (2000) Neural consequences of environmental enrichment. *Nature Reviews Neuroscience* 1, 191–8.

Veissier, I., Buttereworth, A., Bock, B. and Roe, E. (2008) European approaches to ensure good animal welfare. *Applied Animal Behaviour Science* 113, 279–97.

Verkade, T. (1997) *Homeopathy Handbook for Dairy Farming.* Fast Print, Hamilton.

Vertes, R.P. (2004) Memory consolidation in sleep: dream or reality. *Neuron* 44, 135–48.

Walk, R.D. (1958) Visual and visual-motor experience: a replication. *Journal of Comparative and Physiological Psychology* 51, 785–7.

Walsh, R.N. and Cummins, R.A. (1976) The open-field test: a critical review. *Psychological Bulletin* **83**, 482–504.

Watson, C.S., Schaefer, R., White, S.E., Homan, J.H., Fraher, L., Harding, R. and Bocking, A.D. (2002) Effect of intermittent umbilical cord occlusion on fetal respiratory activity and brain adenosine in late-gestation sheep. *Reproduction Fertility and Development* **14**, 35–42.

Webster, A.B. (2004) Welfare implications of avian osteoporosis. *Poultry Science* **83**, 184–92.

Webster, J. (1994) *Animal Welfare: a Cool Eye Towards Eden.* Blackwell Science, Oxford.

Webster, J. (2005a) The assessment and implementation of animal welfare: theory into practice. *Scientific and Technical Review of the Office International des Epizooties* **24**, 723–34.

Webster, J. (2005b) *Animal Welfare: Limping Towards Eden.* Blackwell Science, Oxford.

Weller, R.F. and Cooper, A. (1996) Health status of dairy herds converting from conventional to organic dairy farming. *Veterinary Record* **139**, 141–2.

Weller, R.F. and Bowling, P.J. (2000) Health status of dairy herds in organic farming. *Veterinary Record* **146**, 80–81.

Wells, D.N. and Laible, G. (2007) Cloning and transgenesis to redesign livestock. In *Redesigning Animal Agriculture*, Swain, D.L., Charmley, E., Steel, J.W. and Coffey, S.G. (eds), pp. 94–120. CABI Publishing, Wallingford.

Wells, D.N., Forsyth, J.T., MacMillan, V. and Oback, B. (2004) Review: the health of somatic cell cloned cattle and their offspring. *Cloning Stem Cells* **6**, 101–10.

Welp, T., Rushen, J., Kramer, D.L., Fest-Blanchet, M. and de Passille, A.M.B. (2004) Vigilance as a measure of fear in dairy cattle. *Applied Animal Behaviour Science* **87**, 1–13.

Wemelsfelder, F. (1997a) Life in captivity: its lack of opportunities for variable behaviour. *Applied Animal Behaviour Science* **54**, 67–70.

Wemelsfelder, F. (1997b) The scientific validity of subjective concepts in models of animal welfare. *Applied Animal Behaviour Science* **53**, 75–88.

West, D.M., Bruere, A.N. and Ridler, A.L. (2002) *The Sheep (Health, Disease and Production).* Foundation for Continuing Veterinary Education of the New Zealand Veterinary Association, Massey University, Palmerston North.

Whateley, J., Kilgour, R. and Dalton, D.C. (1974) Behaviour of hill country sheep breeds during farming routines. *Proceeding of the New Zealand Society of Animal Production* **34**, 28–36.

Williams, V.M., Mellor, D.J. and Marbrook, J. (2006) Revision of a scale for assessing the severity of live animal manipulations. *ALTEX (Special Issue)* **23**, 163–9.

Williams, V.M., Dale, A.R., Clarke, N. and Garrett, N.K.G. (2008) Animal abuse and family violence: Survey on the recognition of animal abuse by veterinarians in New Zealand and their understanding of the correlation between animal abuse and human violence. *New Zealand Veterinary Journal* **56**, 21–8.

Williamson, G. and Payne, E.J.A. (1978) *Animal Husbandry in the Tropics.* Longman, London.

Willis, R. (1974) *Man and Beast*. Granada Publishing., London.

Wilson, R.T. (2002) Specific welfare problems associated with working horses. In *The Welfare of the Horse*, Waran, N. (ed.), pp. 203–18. Kluwer Academic Publishing, Dordrecht.

Windsor, R.S. (2004) Cattle disease in Africa. In *Bovine Medicine*, Andrews, A.H. (ed.), pp. 1156–63. Blackwell Science, Oxford.

Winograd, N. (2005) Temperament testing in the age of no-kill. *Sheltering* January/February. www.nokilladvocacycenter.org/pdf/Temperament%20Testing.pdf.

Wolfe, T. (1985) Laboratory animal technicians: their role in stress reduction and human-companion animal bonding. In Symposium on the Human-Companion Animal Bond, Quackenbush, J. and Voith, V.L. (eds). *Veterinary Clinics of North America: Small Animal Practice* **15**, 449–54.

Woodcock, E. (2004) *Effects of Environmental Enrichment on Fundamental Cognitive Processes in Rats and Humans*. PhD thesis, School of Psychology, University of New South Wales.

Woods, P.J., Fiske, A.S. and Ruckelshaus, S.I. (1961) The effects of drives conflicting with exploration on the problem-solving behavior of rats reared in free and restricted environments. *Journal of Comparative and Physiological Psychology* **54**, 167–9.

Würbel, H. (2000) Behaviour and the standardization fallacy. *Nature Genetics* **26**, 263.

Yeates, J.W. and Main, D.C.J. (2008) Assessment of positive welfare: a review. *Veterinary Journal* **175**, 293–300.

Young, R.J. (2003) *Environmental Enrichment for Captive Animals*. Blackwell Science, Oxford.

Zeder, M.A., Bradley, D.G., Emshwiller, E. and Smith, B.D. (2006) *Documenting Domestication*. University of California Press, Berkeley, CA.

Zimbardo, P.G. and Montgomery, K.C. (1957) Effects of "free environment"rearing upon exploratory behavior. *Psychological Reports* **3**, 589–94.

Index

Page numbers in *italics* refer to figures, those in bold refer to tables.